BIRTHING the TAO

Supporting the Incarnating Soul's Development
through Pregnancy or Rebirthing

RANDINE LEWIS

Foreword by Lorie Dechar

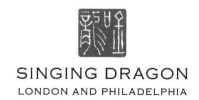

SINGING DRAGON
LONDON AND PHILADELPHIA

First published in Great Britain in 2023 by Singing Dragon,
an imprint of Jessica Kingsley Publishers
Part of John Murray Press

2

A CIP catalogue record for this title is available from the
British Library and the Library of Congress

ISBN 978 1 78775 999 2
eISBN 978 1 83997 003 0

Printed and bound by CPI Group (UK) Ltd, Croydon, CR0 4YY

Jessica Kingsley Publishers' policy is to use papers that are natural, renewable and recyclable
products and made from wood grown in sustainable forests. The logging and manufacturing
processes are expected to conform to the environmental regulations of the country of origin.

Jessica Kingsley Publishers
Carmelite House
50 Victoria Embankment
London EC4Y 0DZ

www.singingdragon.com

John Murray Press
Part of Hodder & Stoughton Limited
An Hachette UK Company

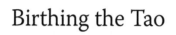

Birthing the Tao

Contents

Foreword

For nearly two decades, I have had the honor and delight of wandering the misty mountains and circuitous pathways of traditional Chinese medicine (TCM) in the company of Dr. Randine Lewis. In fact, I have no doubt that Randine and I have walked the Way together many times before, wearing the garb of hermit healers, mystical midwives, dancing shamans, eccentric wizards, and star-struck alchemists, depending on the era and the place. Yet, wherever, and whenever our pathways cross, we find ourselves in passionate conversation, always searching for a deeper understanding of, in Randine's words, "the mysteries of the origin of life and the laws by which nothing becomes something."

I am deeply grateful to Randine for being an inspiring colleague, a daring and devoted co-traveler and trusted friend. However, the truth is that my gratitude extends far beyond the personal to touch the limits of what I imagine to be the longings of our planet, of Gaia, our mother, and our home. As our planet tumbles wildly through the tumultuous waters of transformation, as our climate veers erratically between fire and flood, as our resources dwindle and our accepted cultural norms collapse, Earth asks us to face the shattering question of how and why we continue to invite new beings to join us here.

Earth calls us to reckon with the toll each one of us takes on her body, the demands each one of us makes on her essences. She asks us to seriously consider the question of why, in the face of climate chaos, rising homelessness, and economic instability, as well as the specter of our own species' extinction, our hearts continue to spill over with celebratory anticipation, excitement, and joy in the presence of conception, gestation, pregnancy, and, most especially, the momentous birth of a child?

Gaia urgently calls us to look deeply, down to the most hidden roots of our own being, and ask, "Just what are we up to when we choose to initiate a new life?" "What are we up to when we employ temperature charts, hormone injections, in vitro fertilization, and egg and sperm donors to coax along a reluctant pregnancy?" "And what are we really doing as practitioners of Chinese medicine when we call on the power of needles, Moxa, Qi Gong, and herbal formulas to urge the ephemeral spark of life to nest, flourish, and grow for nine long months in a woman's womb?"

In response to all these crucial questions, Randine Lewis offers us this book.

What you are holding here in your hands is not a textbook on TCM gynecology and obstetrics, or a cookbook presentation of pre and post IVF procedures. It is not a reference guide for points that can be stimulated to adjust endocrine response, enhance the absorption of nutrients and essences, or encourage the flow of Qi and Blood through the pelvis, although all those benefits may come from the practices and understandings offered within these pages. Rather, this is a book about a radical revisioning of the birth process from a medical condition that requires ongoing quantitative assessments, tracking, and interventions to an awe-inspiring mystery that opens a conduit for a soul to travel from the infinite, unknowable Tao of the divine to the knowable Tao of here and now, the realm of embodied existence.

Birthing the Tao is a book of spells and magic, a book that whispers affirmations in the ears of angels, that asks us to touch each point on a prospective mother's body as if it were the tender bud at the tip of the Tree of Heaven. If you dare to truly immerse yourself in these pages, to take your time in integrating the wisdom offered here, and to actively engage with the questions, meditations, and practices, you will be transformed. You will experience an ontological shift in your perception not only of the birth process but also of your own journey from nothingness into being.

This shift in orientation to our purpose and our responsibility as parents, healers, and humans on a planet with finite resources is, I believe, what Gaia is asking of us now.

To remember the gravitas of the invitation as well as the celebration when the invitation is accepted.

To accept the limitations of our own desires and will, and no matter how far we come in our mastery of the technicalities of conception, gestation, pregnancy, and birth, to remain humble in the presence of a miracle.

To never forget that with each new life we bring to Earth's generous table, we are not just birthing a baby; we are, again and again, giving birth to the Tao.

Lorie Dechar

To the mothers who house the children of tomorrow and their practitioners of fertility, accouchement, and the midwifery sciences. May you always tend to your souls first.

Acknowledgments

My gratitude to Jeffrey Yuen, from whose life-changing classical Taoist teachings I have gleaned much of what inspired this writing; to Claire Wilson of Singing Dragon for the invitation and platform to present this work; and to Stella Osorojos Eisenstein for her immensely helpful editing.

After decades of attempting to answer the age old question of how and why spirits incarnate, I am no closer to the answers. Sue Monk Kidd, in Dance of the Dissident Daughter, offers conception labor and birthing as "metaphors thick with the image and experiences of women (that) offer a body parable of the process of awakening." And in further describing this mysterious parable, she describes pregnancy as telling us "things we need to know about the way awakening works—the slow, unfolding, sometimes hidden, always expanding nature of it, the inevitable queasiness, the need to nurture and attend to what inhabits us, the uncertainty about the outcome, the fearful knowing that once we bring the new consciousness forth, our lives will never be the same." Together we'll delve into the Taoist narrative and its implications for fertility, gestation, and birthing higher levels of consciousness into being; all of which are intertwined in the ancient depictions of how spirit emerges through matter, in matter, as matter.

Introduction

As acorns bounce like popcorn across my deck, I ponder how these little capped marvels could possibly become the shady oak trees surrounding my cabin; but really—I don't want to know how. I'd rather remain in awe *that* an acorn somehow becomes a shade tree. Mysteries are far more compelling.

A newly pregnant patient anxiously tells me that she has been spotting pink, watery blood. Treatment begins as my hand rests on her wrist, my touch conveying that I feel her fear as I notice her hollow Spleen pulse is not ascending. I use a Taoist metaphor and tell her, "When the star seeds of this spirit were scooped up by the Big Dipper and poured into your baby's heart, its pure light was captured by the essence of Water. Like the banks of a river, your Earth element must hold on to this celestial being, and your Spleen is straining to keep up with this miracle in creation. See if you can find a place within where your worry can merge with trust." As I gently insert needles, she closes her eyes, her heart rate slows down, her breath deepens, and she relaxes into the peace this story provides. She has just met her child in the place where the acorn grows.

Gestation isn't meant to be figured out; it is not a medical condition but a mystery—far too vast to comprehend. Hence, the Taoists used a mythic model to describe how the soul is programmed in the "dark womb" with its constitution, temperament, and what it will need to survive and thrive in its upcoming life. Immersing in the story of the embryo's journey, we will come to comprehend the energetic physiology going on beneath the surface and how it affects the mother, and address any symptoms with Chinese medicine, while never losing sight of the fact that we are tending to an embodying soul.

All true healing brings us to a deeper place within ourselves. Popular self-help techniques approach healing like surgical intervention—figure out what's wrong, so it can be fixed, modified, or discarded. This is like cutting apart the acorn to inspect its insides in order to make it grow. Merely analyzing and trying to modify the form will never allow us to move the spirits, which the *Su Wen* (Huang Di's *Inner Classic*) insists must be done. As practitioners, we must access the place of the unborn potential, like preparing the ground for the acorn to sprout in the dark womb of source.

The Secret of the Golden Flower by Richard Wilhelm tells us that when the dark is at rest, the light begins to move, where a new potential emerges out of the dark. The most radical healing often occurs beyond diagnosis and intervention. Patterns provide guideposts that can lead us deeper into the power of Yin, our own dark and mysterious recesses at one with the source. The ancestral beginning is darkness waiting to be lit. When our minds are completely at rest and surrendered to the mystery, a deeper part of us, like a distant echo, responds, inviting the soul of our true selves to spring forth. The light begins to move and an unrealized possibility arises.

The majority of my professional career has been spent in the field of fertility, yet my deepest passion has never been about managing pregnancy or birthing babies. I've always been intrigued, however, with the mystery of the origin of life and the laws by which nothing becomes something. After studying Chinese medicine, my unceasing inquiries about how spirit infuses itself into form met the mystery of the Tao, through various writings—some well known, some more esoteric—and I couldn't get enough. I had been treating fertility for years when I first heard 88th generation Taoist Priest Jeffrey Yuen. While his unsurpassed knowledge of medicine blew my heart and mind, his teachings describing the Taoist origin and meaning of life were like poetry that soothed the restlessness of my soul. While I have been deeply moved by him and other teachers, this work is my own interpretation. Quotes without sources are my own words.

While I considered myself well versed in fertility strategies, personal and clinical experiences sometimes defied the best my mind could come up with. You may know what that's like—you do everything you can and then come to the edge of what you know. At the top of my game, I'd seem to stall; but that, I found out, was the portal—the surrender point into the unborn. If I didn't react from fear of not knowing or getting it right, and instead let go into the pause of the unknown, another gear would sometimes kick in and Shen would take over. Same points, same techniques, but suddenly everything would lighten up, charged with a new glow that seemed to come from beyond. And the patients' spirits would be moved.

I continued to learn more—we have to in our field—but I also learned to empty my head and hit my knees more often. I tried to teach my patients the same. The more I worked in the realm of the unborn, it seemed an immediate and eternal presence would infuse itself into the most intimate moments, and the patients would be changed. While I might not be able to explain or recreate what had just happened, it seemed there were some commonalities—those more prone to miracles were the ones who were able to relinquish control so the required shifts in consciousness could take place. When the spirits were moved, the Qi would follow. This isn't "magic;" it is the result of contemplation. The key to expertise in our medicine only begins with how much Chinese medicine we know. True mastery comes when the practitioner begins to know herself and her source. And this comes from deep, ongoing, soul-searching cultivation practices.

After decades of attempting to answer the age-old question of how and why spirits incarnate, I am no closer to the answers. But together we'll delve into the Taoist narrative and its implications for fertility, gestation, and birthing higher levels of consciousness into being, all of which are intertwined in the ancient depictions of how spirit emerges through matter, in matter, as matter.

From our shamanic roots, *Birthing the Tao* is really Taoist embryology in a nutshell, providing a landscape of the soul's journey into existence throughout the themes that correspond with the ten lunar months of pregnancy. Each has its dominant energetic element, which determines how the fetus receives its curriculum, unique temperament, and the challenges it will need to fulfill its destiny. As we weave biomedical manifestations into a Taoist narrative of the soul's passage through the three thematic trimesters of pregnancy, we'll reveal how its transition from one stage to another impacts the mother and explains many of her health concerns. As practitioners learn to appreciate the profoundly important energetics of the developing fetus, they can make sense of many of the patients' symptoms and their Chinese medical energetic corollaries.

The Western-based medical models, and even TCM sometimes, still treat pregnancy anxiously, marinating mother and baby in stress hormones. When we go to the doctor to check if everything's okay, it may seem like prudence, but behind it lurks the fear that something might be wrong, and fear weakens the Essence and constricts uterine blood flow. Ongoing maternal fear increases the output of stress hormones, which maximizes the baby's stress response, shifting fetal neurological development. Their brainstems get heightened attention at the expense of higher cognitive maturation. Treating issues once they have manifested is the lowest grade of medicine; rarely does it reach the root from which all imbalances arise—being out of harmony with one's true nature. Think about it—going to the clinic to get our blood work drawn or our pulse taken to make sure we aren't manifesting some hidden disease state makes for more fearful and lazy patients, who put their health in the hands of someone else. While prevention of disease states is favorable, avoidance of sickness is not the highest grade of medicine either; that belongs to the Pericardium's protective function. The upper grade of medicine brings one to a place of honoring one's own divinity—I love my life too much to allow myself to become ill, so I will radically attend to my own health and wellbeing.

Most pregnant women fear something will go awry with their pregnancy and their baby might not be okay. The entire field of obstetrics is based on what might go wrong—ultrasounds to make sure all of the parts measure the right size at the right time; screenings for genetic abnormalities—the entire process is on the lookout for pathology. Disempowered patients with no prenatal preparation hold their breath until the amniocentesis comes back normal, eat whatever they want until they develop gestational diabetes, and exercise as they did or didn't before pregnancy, becoming plagued with back pain, edema, and candidates for C-sections.

What if, while we let obstetricians run their standard tests, we were to assume the pregnancy and its baby were just fine, being nurtured by the long line of mothers who have gestated before us, all the way back to the very first mother, the primordial ancestor, and instead tended to our own souls? Taking pregnancy out of a fear-based model of symptom resolution and replacing it with a broader and deeper understanding, practitioners will learn how to support patients from before conception through birth, calmly tending to each of the soul's developmental milestones during pregnancy and addressing the mothers' most common concerns as they come along. And all the while we'll remind them of the story of their own life, their own roots, as mother and baby go through this journey together.

Science is now proving that unresolved physical, emotional, mental, and spiritual impediments become hurdles to the health and growth of a new life. When an individual addresses all aspects of their wellbeing before they take on the life of another, they relieve their children from inheriting the burdens of their unresolved past, inviting them to manifest their highest potential. A new life thrives in a good physical home, free of stress, toxins, and emotional upset. And when a healthy pregnancy is achieved, very little intervention is required. Preparing the soil beforehand helps a plant thrive far more than trying to manipulate its growth once above ground. Pregnancy should be a time of easing oneself deeper and deeper into the process of welcoming ourselves and any new life we bring forth into the world.

While *Birthing the Tao* may borrow quotes from various classical texts, it will not simply report them, but make the wisdom tradition applicable to the modern-day understanding of physiology, psychology, and the meaning of life. It is my intention to take the teachings of the Taoist origins of Chinese medicine, much of which come from an oral tradition, and delve deeper than the disempowering focus on symptom resolution, to instead nourish the very roots of our source in a very practical way that resonates with our modern intellect. When we are in the realm of the soul's potential, we have access to prenatal energies from which all of our creative energies in life arise.

The Taoist pregnancy narrative provides a map for the soul of the practitioner and patient, where they can journey together in the mysterious land where hope is made manifest. Tools are provided for the practitioner to develop richer and more comprehensive acupuncture and herbal treatment strategies specific to each patient. Queries are offered for the mother to connect with her seedling, along with meditative, dietary, and lifestyle suggestions, and self-inquiry worksheets applicable for each month of pregnancy. Whether the patient is gestating another being or her true self, these methods will help the mother connect with the cocooned inner soul to encourage a healthy and robust pregnancy, delivery, and birth experience. We will delve into the questions the Taoists asked, not with the attempt to answer, but to live, into the meaning of this mysterious life. In today's world we need more wonder, more hope, less fear. We need more soul, especially in the treatment room.

As we pave the way for the souls of tomorrow, we become as guides that honor the enormity of the soul's sacred journey through pregnancy. In *Song of Myself*, Walt Whitman describes how generations of cosmic and evolutionary forces are employed to complete the embryo until *on this spot I stand with my robust soul*. Now we can begin to understand why at birth, the child is already a year old.

> *Before I was born out of my mother generations guided me,*
>
> *my embryo has never been torpid, nothing could overlay it.*

For it the nebula cohered to an orb,
the long slow strata piled to rest it on,
vast vegetables gave it sustenance,

monstrous sauroids transported it in their mouths and deposited it with care.
All forces have been steadily employ'd to complete and delight me,
now on this spot I stand with my robust soul.

—Walt Whitman, "Song of Myself, 44"

Prologue

Long ago, before the Tao birthed itself into its myriad manifestations, the entire universal flux of all that is swirled within an egg-shaped cosmic cloud, the birthplace of galaxies. Tens of thousands of years it swirled, building up pressure until it exploded into an enormous being called Pangu. As the giant emerged, it went about dividing things: that which was light evaporated to become sky, that which was negative sank to become earth, and Pangu stood in between, getting lost in the separation. The eyes took their place as the sun and moon; the breath became the wind; body turned into mountains; and blood flowed as rivers. The skull domed the sky, and hair adorned the heavens with stars. The flesh became earth covered with skin of grasses and flowers, upon which two-legged critters whose head reached toward heaven and whose feet held the earth lived. They, like Pangu, held the power of creation within them, although they did not know it. They first had to journey through their inner terrain until they found and lived their true destinies.

The Taoists view the human body as a microcosm of this celestial realm. Just as a human being is a microcosm of the macrocosm, we each contain an entire universe—whose inner hills and valleys are inhabited by resident deities and demons, and whose cosmic command post resides in the center of the head amidst the Nine Peaks of the Immortals where Big Shen—our reflection of the eternal light of universal intelligence—resides.

Humans also went about separating. They called the bright principle Yang; by it they could see, making them feel in control—therefore the light was revered. The dark principle they called Yin; it was black and mysterious and made them feel vulnerable. Although Yin provided rest, it was feared and eventually dishonored. The Yin and Yang principles in nature became the Yin and Yang principles in the human body. We often fear our own dark and unknown depths in preference for that which is already familiar, but we reproduce the entire holon and wonder why our creations show up with that which we abhor in ourselves.

PART I

PREPARING THE PALACE

Basics of Gynecological Obstetrics

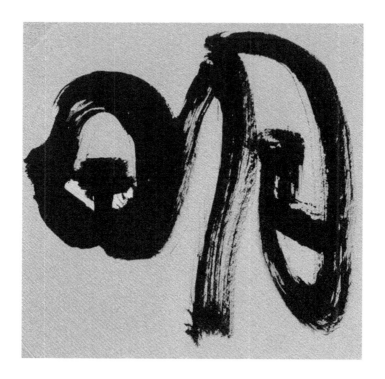

CHAPTER 1

The Origin

THE MIRACLE OF MANIFESTATION

In the beginning was the Tao.
It gives birth to all beings,
nourishes them, maintains them, cares for them,
comforts them, protects them,
and takes them back to itself.
This is its story.
The story of you.

Fertility and pregnancy are often viewed strictly as a physical phenomenon where sperm penetrates an egg, develops into an embryo, and grows into a fetus, which, in the absence of complications, will be birthed as a baby. While the physical focus is the most common narrative discussed in almost every book on pregnancy, it isn't the only view; in fact, to carry a baby used to be held as nothing short of a miracle. Yes, we like to know how big the uterus is supposed to be and what phases of physical development the fetus should be going through. We like to know what type of symptoms to expect, too. Yet most women feel that there is a more miraculous process going on beneath the surface that isn't limited to size and symptoms, a great undertaking that opens the heart into the wonder and reverence for creation itself.

Somehow, that which is not provokes a longing that then becomes that which is. While we can't (and nor do we want to) rationally explain this phenomenon, pregnancy can provide a beautifully poetic metaphor for how and why life manifests, as well as its purpose. The Huainanzi says, *To find the origin, trace back the manifestation.* No matter where we are in our life journey, we can trace our way back to our source; we don't ever have to lose this sense of wonder and awe.

When the coming of life was viewed as a miracle, humanity seemed to be more connected to our deep, dark origin—less lost in fascination for its manifestations. While our feet walked in the physical world, we simultaneously attended to the spirit. In my years ushering fertility patients toward some type of healing, there seemed to be two intertwining and unmet desires. The first one—the one that brought them to seek help—was the desire for a child. This is one of the strongest urges in life. Kahlil Gibran, in *The Prophet*, describes it in his poem "On Children" as *Life's longing for itself.* There seems to be an otherworldly force behind this need—which can often take over a woman's life. At times her very survival seems to depend upon whether a baby would manifest through her body and into her life. But behind this I perceived a more nebulous and less urgent need to know the purpose of her life. I found it interesting that the intense demand for a baby superseded the very reason for one's own existence. Having contemplated this conundrum personally as well, I wondered if we might just have it backwards. Those who are complete and harmonious within themselves are certainly in a better place to bring forth more harmony and completion than those who don't know who they are. While we might argue that knowing oneself is not a prerequisite for bearing children, we are in a very different world today than our Chinese forebears, and it certainly can provide an advantage.

Everyone who has been with child knows that they are carrying a miracle. The perhaps overused phrase "pregnant with possibility" conveys a feeling of the immensity of creation, coming through each child. All of Heaven and Earth are contained in this little being, growing according to rules we can never fully understand with our finite minds. Yet here, in the womb of the Mysterious Mother, whom we channel, life has chosen to manifest. Wow.

> You may ask, "Whose child is it?"—but I cannot say.
> This child was here before the Great Ancestor.
>
> —*Tao Te Ching (Book of the Way), Chapter 4*

Perhaps the longing for life is the closest we can come to experiencing the raw amazement that we are here, right now, through this instrument of creation itself. We are each here for a reason that supersedes anything that we do in life—having children, healing others, saving the world—we are here to discover through our personal life story the very purpose for our being. It is to find our way home, to our true selves, to our destination, which is also our origin. Once upon an eternal time called now, it just didn't make sense to bring forth another before we brought ourselves forth fully, in all of our glory.

Just like the strength of life's longing for itself, if we go against this internal dictate, we ail. We go through life in a contracted state, feeling like something is missing, something isn't quite right. This sense of something missing can be projected upon our life situation and we look for substitutes—a child, a partner, a new job or home, another child—to make us feel whole. But no outside thing will ever fill what can only be recovered within. Chapter 1 of the *Su Wen* says of the saints of high antiquity:

> In peaceful calm, void and emptiness, the authentic Qi flows easily. Essences and spirits are kept within. How could illnesses arise? They restrained their wills and diminished desire. At peace in their heart, they felt no fear. They worked hard and were not exhausted. The Qi followed a regular course. Each followed their desire and all were content.

Desires squander our inner treasures of Qi externally, rendering us ever discontent. Yet the sages followed their desires and were content. What gives? First of all, pure desires in alignment with the destiny of one's soul will be fulfilled. It's what spurs the will to move us forward. It seems that going *outside* of ourselves to fill what's missing is what doesn't work. Hope is an inner force, a radiating movement directing us toward something higher from within. Our deepest trauma is being torn from our cosmic womb, and our highest longing is for reunion with our origin. That's an inside job. The separate egoic sense of self is not meant to be our end point; unity is both our birthright and our destiny. And letting go of our finite sense of who we think we have been precedes becoming who we were meant to be.

When Heaven unites with Earth to create a human being, it etches a set of laws into our very being, which subtly, but very clearly, urges us to discover why we are here.

Sometimes it appears that the great and majestic cosmic order of Heaven goes on indifferent to our little human endeavors. Yet Heaven isn't a place, but a divine power through which our lives are directed. Down here, in the divine drama of human life, where we breed and bleed, we need meaning. We need to know that we are not merely insignificant blips on the screen of eternity, accidental and directionless, fighting for survival, an offspring or two, and a few years of pleasure until we meet our final demise. We will continue to feel the ache of our deficiency until the alchemy of coming to know the quantum reality of our true nature happens.

We often view babies as fresh, cooing, powdery-smelling bundles meant to be cuddled and nurtured until they grow up, get good jobs, and then take care of their elderly parents. However, the sweet potential of a newly entering baby disguises an enormous truth about the push behind the cycle of life. Birth doesn't just happen one time at the beginning where death marks finality at the end. Death and rebirth are an ongoing process throughout life, which begins as soon as a cell divides. When an egg takes a sperm in, life as a seed is over. A fetus must die to life in utero so it may be labored into the world. We lay down our lives as children in order to enter into adulthood, expiring through various phases of human growth and development until we are finally birthed back into the Tao. Let's start with the understanding that from the moment nothing becomes something, all of life reverberates with this eternal affair of becoming and unbecoming.

Our souls are the very internal blueprint that tell our hearts and minds who and what we are and propel us toward the Tao's whole-making function. When we encounter anything at that level, we can't help but love, respect, and protect it. Our true selves are very childlike, yet also supernaturally wise. It is said that the purpose of life is to find and connect with this internal guidance system, and when we recover the sense of heavenly direction, it will lead us to our destiny. Not as some externally oriented destination, but more like the guiding principle of entelechy, which takes the soul to its fruition the way an acorn unfolds into an oak tree. If we cultivate this awareness and shine our own beacon of awareness to our origin, a brightness of spirit shines forth, directing our lives from within. First, however, we often have to go through the necessary process of cleaning up the constitution as the light reveals all kinds of shadows and inauthentic substitutes. But as we continue to correct our course, this treasure can be intensified and accompany us as we venture through life and find our way back to the Tao. Like the wise old baby represented by Lao Tzu's enlightenment, we are the ones we've been searching for. And the map for the soul is woven together as the star seeds dance within the earthly womb of the Mysterious Mother during the process of pregnancy itself. It is there within us all the time, just waiting for our eyes to shift inward—toward Heaven.

As the microcosm is a hologram of the macrocosm, our individual stories are woven inside of the great universal story. The threads that link them together are provided by myths—archetypal representations of deeper eternal truths that we feel within our bones. Here's how it all begins.

Conception

> Born of Heaven is my virtue,
> born of Earth is my Qi.
> Heavenly Virtue, Earthly Qi wrestle,
> giving rise to the human.
> Thus the primal substance evolving to become the human body is known as Jing.
> Yin and Yang unite to produce the movement of life known as Shen.

—Ling Shu (Spiritual Pivot, The Ancient Classic on Needle Therapy), Chapter 8

Through the ecstatic and ritual act of merging in love, an electromagnetic field is created. Of course, pregnancies can also result from unwanted sexual encounters or in an embryology laboratory, each of which has its own energy. Yet we all have the capacity to shift the energetic field of any environment in which we find ourselves.

Let's say we're in an atmosphere created by love and devotion between a man and a woman. Each has a different arousal response; the Lung–Kidney axis is dominant in a male, while the Heart–Kidney axis dominates the female response. In both, the Liver channel, which runs through the genitals, is activated. The Mawangdui silk manuscript, written prior to 168 BCE, describes the following: "To generate a human being, the man has to enter into the obscure darkness and exit from the obscure darkness; thus begins the process of making a human." In the ritual act of sexual intercourse, the essence that is located in the pelvic region becomes excited. The couple's breath rate increases, and their embodied, corporeal souls become enlivened. In one wondrous moment out of time, the sexual fluids combine, from which the friction of opposing Yin and Yang forces creates a highly charged and specific vibration, which invokes and draws down a third energy, precipitated from the heavenly realms. The Jing embrace, and the three become one.

Jing

> No form of the great ancestor of matter.
> No sound is the great ancestor of the voice.
> The child (of no form) is light.
> The grandchild (of no form) is water.
> All are created from no form.
> Light can be seen, it cannot be grasped.
> Water can be molded, it cannot be destroyed.
> Therefore of all things that have matter, nothing is more respectable than water.
>
> —*Huai Nan Zi, Chapter 2*

Jing is associated with our basic morphology. This vital is defined as a precious, high-quality substance of cosmic vitality, which gives all beings their aliveness. Yet, only fiery, expansive Shen has the power to animate, so it first has to fuse with watery Jing. Just as sunlight isn't perceptible until it is reflected by form, Shen—a light that penetrates from above—can't be realized without Jing, and Jing can't burst open with its inherent aliveness without Shen. Qi is the medium by which the original life-giving spirit materializes into, or appears as, Jing. In fact, Jing is seen as a Yin, a concentrated state of Qi that allows form to be enlivened as the very basis of life.

Zhuang Zi says that the beginnings blend in a dark and unclear place, and that absolute Jing has no form. It is the underlying non-divisible substratum of every living being that has to go through a few steps in order to come about. Yuan (source) defines the underlying creative life principles from the cosmos that sparks the spirit of creation into existence. First, the purity of Heaven's undifferentiated light has to slow its vibration down to the level of consciousness so Yuan Shen (original spirit) can condense into Yuan (source) Qi (the animating breath of Life), which then precipitates into Yuan Jing, which is still prior to materialization. On the verge of becoming matter, Yuan Jing then coalesces into "rough" Jing, which contains the subtle pattern of life, emerging between the

Kidneys as the source of Yuan Qi, which will be distributed unevenly through the back Shu points to give the new being its unique constitutional makeup. Yuan Jing, like a wave on the verge of becoming a particle, remains pure potential throughout life as Tian Ji (threads that connect us to Heaven). From the dark origin, these silken threads weave a mysterious connection from the source and hook onto the Ming at Du 4 Mingmen (Gate of Destiny). When we have walked the path toward our true destiny, the realms of the subtle are accessible through our Heart-Mind and we gain conscious access to the process by which the macrocosm perpetually becomes the microcosm. These threads of Heaven hanging down from Heaven are imperceptible to the ordinary human whose eyes are set on worldly things, but the realized being is able to connect to the Tian Ji within, and work the shuttle of Heaven's loom.

Yuan Qi transforms Jing into Kidney Qi. While Jing, which contain our heavenly mandate, are the coarsest of the three Treasures (Jing, Qi, and Shen), we must do our best not to contaminate them with rough living, mental agitation, and poor eating, which deplete Kidney Qi. Through meditation and cultivation we can concentrate them and keep them as pure as possible.

Fertilization

The Ming dynasty physician Zhang Jie Bin, author of the Leijing (類經) and Jingyue quanshu (景岳全書) described how the united Yin and Yang essences of the parents intertwine to form the Heart-Mind. If we combine the views of quantum physics with the mystic wisdom traditions, we could say that Life is a disturbance in the field of Shen, which comes into being centripetally. In the absolute Yin of the void where there is nothing but the pure inertia of the Mysterious Mother, the hand of Shang Di, the supreme deity of the Tao, somehow stirs a miraculous force to orbit inward until it begins to consolidate into a nucleus. As the universe enfleshes itself at the moment of conception, the strands of materiality provided by the parents' Jing wrap themselves up with the cosmic contribution, including any residue of past incarnations, which is then swirled together and captured in the embrace of the Quintessential Spirit. The star seeds of the eternal spirit pull inward like a tornado, coiling into a center vacuum that contains the energies of contraction and desire, now as a corporeal (Po) soul seeking aliveness. A snapshot of the entire cosmos at this specific moment in space-time is simultaneously captured, scooped up by the Big Dipper, and poured into the core of the fertilized egg.

The fused Jing serve as a divining rod through which this cosmic storm finds a path into this dimension. Like a lightning bolt from Heaven, the original pure light of spirit is captured in earthly form, endowing it with human intelligence, consciousness, and the essence of a unique sense of self. This one cell contains the immense push whereby Yuan Shen (original spirit) became Yuan Qi (breath of Life), Yuan Jing, and Jing—the source energies that provide the polarity by which cellular division will proceed toward its ultimate destiny (Ming). We are still at the formation of the first cell.

This entire cosmic symphony of star dust becoming human goes on within the delicate fronds of the fallopian tubes where union of egg and sperm yields a single cell called a zygote (Greek for "yoked"), which holds the power of this Yin and Yang polarity with 23 chromosomes from each parent uniting, for about a day. If Life wishes to continue beyond the zygote phase, and if the Essence can hold its force, within 24 to 36 hours, the cell will divide.

The origin

Before our body existed,
one energy was already there.
Like jade, more lustrous as it's polished,
like gold, brighter as it's refined.
Sweep clear the ocean of birth and death,
stay firm by the door of total mastery.
A particle at the point of open awareness,
the gentle firing is warm.

—Sun Bu'er, "Immortal Woman"

The original penetrating (Chong) meridian carries our direct mandate from Heaven. It represents the polarity established in each cell and the Tai Qi pole from the top of our head to the tip of the coccyx, which holds our original decree from the powers of creation, and through which we can be reawakened to our reason for being. Only the Heart has the ability to perceive the subtle threads of heaven that come from the center primordial penetrating meridian. Taoist Immortal Women like Sun Bu'er recited spiritual poetry with enchanting birth and rebirthing metaphors to coax us back to the source:

> *Before our body existed, one energy was already there.*
> *The beginning of the sustenance of life is all Yin and Yang.*
> *At the point where the womb breath is continuous, you should*
> *distinguish the beginnings of movement and stillness...*

(From Immortal Sisters *Secret Teachings of Taoist Women*, Thomas Cleary, North Atlantic Books 1996)

When we live according to externals, we tend to be tangentially thrown around by the circumstances in our lives, always at the mercy of something or someone else. Usually our states of mind are not only informed by *but are also dictated* by the worldly events, rather than being informed and anchored by our central core, which always belongs to Heaven and therefore contains its unconditional power. The *Huai Nan Zi* speaks of two heavenly deities that took hold of the handles of the Tao and stood at the center, transforming the four directions. The highest use of our will is to inhabit this universal power at the center of our dualistic being and bring its unitive authority into all facets of our world.

Most of us intuit we are not a mere culmination of historic events in time beginning with birth and ending with death. We are not solely physical; nor are we just swirling mental constructs of thoughts and memories. We are not even limited by our hopes and dreams. There's something indefinably more that is witness to it all. When we find and live from the center of our being, that which holds the eternal meaning of our own existence, life becomes synchronous and resonant. We don't have to try so hard to arrange exteriors to suit us—it naturally flowers into being with a power that the personal will could never muster. We are living from the soul.

The soul

Most traditions depict the soul as that unseeable force that links us with the origin of all. Michael Meade describes the soul as the light concealed in darkness, the divine connection hidden in the heart of each individual and the secret way to hidden unity of the world. It's simultaneously us, and yet not limited to us, and while perceivable to the heart, it isn't measurable with the senses. Hence, we use myths and archetypes to convey its properties. There is no system as complex as the Chinese tradition's rich use of metaphors to describe the multi-faceted dimensions of the spirit, embodying as soul. We begin with one Universal Spirit—Big Shen—that divides into two Yin and Yang counterparts, Shen and Ling. Then arise three divisions of the soul in the body, and five elemental spirits, of which the ethereal and corporeal souls are further separated into ten divisions. Ten represents unity and completion, where the one is in the many and eternity is in each thing.

The One

The unfathomable Tao, the dark and obscure mystery, gives birth to One, the primordial and indivisible unity that underlies all things. Yet unity has no form; as soon as One comes into being, so does the Two, the Three, and the myriad things. In our model, the cosmic Big Shen (before it identifies with an individual self) represents the One. As envoys from Heaven, the Shen are always pure and untainted by life, retaining the pure Yang force of the eternal One that they extend into this existence.

The Two

One can't maintain its oneness in the manifest world that operates according to duality, and so must have polarity. Once Shen embodies through Jing, its Yin aspect is called Ling, meaning the divine state through which the power of the spirit animates the physical. The Chinese character for Ling 靈 is composed of raindrops falling from Heaven above two priestesses performing a ritual dance to effect changes in nature. Ling is the feminine aspect of spirit, ascribed to women because theirs were the bodies through which the souls enter existence, and were therefore seen as closer to creation. Like the moon reflecting the sun, Ling mirrors Shen through the process of embodiment as the vibration caused by atmospheric changes during sexual union attracts precipitation down from the heavenly realms to generate a new human being.

Yes, we do carry the powers of creation within us. Yet it seems the spirits do not respond to the endless desires of our minds. We can't make it rain or produce children on demand simply because we intend them, no matter how hard we cogitate. To indulge our individual desires upsets the cosmic order and only creates disorder. The Taoist sages used rituals to raise their vibratory level to create changes first and foremost within themselves. Only then were they capable of appealing to the powers of Heaven because through these rituals the priestess was capable of moving beyond the confines of the limited and willful egoic self, which—face it—is pretty much impotent. The ego takes energy to sustain, and is thus incapable of giving rise to positive, life-supporting endeavors. The earliest Chinese medicine was practiced by female shamans; it was not an intellectual pursuit, but a connection to the Spirits. The ritual dances they performed used the most efficient geometrical movement in nature—spirals—to release the exterior self and inhabit the central core, the primordial penetrating meridian, so the universal power could act through the individual emptied of its selfish whims. The sage doesn't imagine that she can improve upon the natural course of things according to heaven. She accepts them, and does not compete with them. As she follows the natural order of Heaven, she aligns with its power within her. A new possibility arises.

The Three

As the original spirit (Yuan Shen) incarnates as the eternal soul (Shen Xian) and divides into Yin and Yang, it distributes its spiritual power through three Dan Tiens or power centers that retain their subtle influences to guide one on their spiritual journey through earthly life. Contained in the bony cavities of the pelvis, the thorax, and the skull, they greatly impact our posture, which cannot be separated from our perception of and response to life. When we change our perception, our posture changes:

- The lower Dan Tien that resides just below the navel is associated with Jing; it powers the physical instinct and kinetic movement throughout the body. Male Qi Gong masters focus their energy inside the lower Dan Tien. Psychically, it governs the underworld, which we might call the raw power of Eros. Full of fire and not yet wise, it propels us to meet our basic physical urges. This corresponds to the basic foundational substance of the first trimester, and establishes our identification with the body and anchors the other energies.
- The middle Dan Tien, whose vibration occupies the center of the Heart, regulates the Qi by integrating our experiences, establishes our sovereignty, and governs our ability to interact and empathically communicate

with others. Female Qi Gong masters focus on this power center, which adjusts the tension between the inner dictates of our original spirit and the struggle to conform to the rules, desires, and comforts of the exteriorly made acquired personality. Placed between the pull of the lower urges and the upper realms, the middle Dan Tien programs the Shen in the second trimester, which establishes our identification with the mind and emotions.

- The light of the upper Dan Tien dwells behind the center of the two eyebrows where it communes directly with the cosmic Big Shen, receiving intuitive guidance toward spiritual growth and ultimate awakening to its true illumined nature. The upper Dan Tien represents the mind's power to differentiate between dense activities that pull us into reactivity, where we remain trapped by earthly existence, and those that can propel us beyond our habitual gravitational pull, reaching toward our heavenly home to connect with the reality of the spirits of the cosmos. Our final programming is here in the third trimester, which provides the potential to identify with spirit.

These three power centers provide the exchange between the coarser energies of Jing in the lower Dan Tien, which are transformed by Qi in the middle Dan Tien into Shen in the upper Dan Tien. Babies enter life almost pure Jing. If we are living according to the mandates of Heaven, life will be spent redeeming Shen from Jing through the medium of Qi. And ideally, at the end of our days, the brightness of spirit (Shen Ming) will shine through our entire earthly form, the darkness will dazzle, and our step will be lifted just a few inches off the ground.

The Five

Five spirits describe different facets of the soul or aspects of the psyche; how the pure light of Heaven is diffracted through the five Yin organs, giving us our unique temperament and the organizing principles of our mind. Prenatally, the first three spirits (Shen, Hun, and Po) set the stage for life, while the last two (Yi and Zhi) are programmed postnatally by how we respond to life, based upon what we allow to inhabit our Hearts and minds.

While Shen comes and goes in its movements
there emerges the function of perception/consciousness known as Hun.

> With Jing Qi together it enters and exits thus producing
> the function of mobility known as Po.
>
> —*Ling Shu, Chapter 8*

Shen 神 describe how the radiant astrological influences extended from heaven above are infused into this earthly existence. Pure, infinite, cosmic light, Shen provide a luminous vitality by which the will of Heaven becomes known through the mind and intellect. Shen is the consciousness of knowing one's existence; through Shen, one is conscious of all things perceived through the mind or senses, and Shen endows insight. This Fire energy that enlivens the psyche resides in the Heart, which provides a quiet and tranquil home for the spirits. While they remain pure and unchanged, Shen are the means by which all transformation occurs.

Hun 魂—The Yang aspect of the soul is made up of the three Hun or cloud spirits: rarefied supernatural Qi referred to collectively as the Ethereal Soul. The Hun follow the Shen and report to Heaven every 60 days on the spiritual progress the individual is making on their life journey. The Hun, which belong both to heaven and us, survive the body, and like a mist flow back to Heaven when this manifest form of existence is over. In life, the Hun describe our ability to dream, and aspire to achieve our visions. The Hun come and go, and their movement is upward. They are rooted in the Liver, and belong to the Wood element, and the easterly direction.

Po 魄—The white spirits of the corporeal soul are associated with the physical body and the white bones of death and resurrection. The Yin, earthbound Po represent the polarity of contraction and expansion by which the soul takes somatic manifestation. The Po are depicted as ghostly presences that need tangibility, so they look for a physical doorway, which they find and enter at Po Men, at the base of the coccyx where the Du Mai (Governing Meridian) begins. There are seven themes that arise as Po "issues," life lessons that are stored in the physical body primarily beneath the surface of our conscious awareness. When they are activated and become conscious, we have the opportunity to recognize and befriend them, where they become powerful allies of transformation. As our lessons are learned, they may depart, or they may continue to accompany us in deeper alchemical journeys. The Po belong to the Lung, the Metal element, and the western direction. The Hun and Po rely on and communicate with one another throughout life. At death, when the Hun ascend to Heaven, the Po descend to be buried in the Earth.

Yi 意 depicts the harmonic vibration produced by one's Heart, the particular resonance that guides our thoughts, words, and actions into manifestation. Yi refers to the process by which the deepest part of our being, the very root of our mind, gives us our conscious bearings. This disposition of awareness allows us to discern what we allow into the Heart, and becomes the means by which we each uniquely perceive situations, and understand and express ourselves in life to create the fabric of our reality. Belonging to the Spleen and governed by the Earth element, the function of Yi is the Qi through which the Heart applies itself to formulate thoughts, beliefs, and ideas. The power of awareness precedes the mental forms it takes. When the Heart applies itself through Yi, we have intention. So, while intention has the power of the Heart behind it, it is our very ability to be aware that allows the spirits to act when we are in alignment with Heaven and nature. Desirous thoughts that covet a particular thing do not have the same strength, as they live in the realm of manifest mental forms, and when the mind overly focuses on them, it disperses the Qi outward, draining our resources. When we deepen our awareness to the energy field beneath the particulates of thought forms, Yi is the power that projects the hologram of our physical reality, where the divine intelligence wordlessly reveals our true nature in all that the mind contacts.

Zhi 志—A shoot emerging from the depths of the heart through which life and its will to survive arises as an instinctual power that ignites the flame of organic processes. The Zhi spirit represents how we feel about our deepest selves; it provides the basis that orients the Will, and gives one a sense of ambition and purpose. Zhi is the spirit of the Kidneys, which belongs to the Water element, ever seeking deeper furrows to anchor our drives in the ongoing process of ensoulment. When Yi becomes permanent, we speak of Zhi, a strong orientation that keeps us on course, like a rudder that guides and gives continuity to our moment-to-moment movements. Together, the Yi and Zhi make up the disposition that rules one's inner life. When Yi roots itself in Zhi, all of the Heart-Mind functions are in alignment, giving us the continuity we will need to access our deepest wisdom.

While we can devote our Wills to almost anything, pure or impure, the highest drive we can aspire to is to discover the origin of our own true nature. This Will is so aligned with Heaven that it is said to originate from the source, like an echo of the Mysterious Mother beckoning, "Come find me; there you will find yourself." And we must follow. This is what is spoken of as completion.

The Ten

The Taoist soul is made up of almost infinite representations of how vast we really are, actual microcosms of the boundless cosmos. From the initial intent to manifest, we are here by universal design, and with a very specific purpose: we are here to learn. Not to collect data as in a classroom, but as star seeds earthed into being on a mission. We souls are unleashed into the world with a lesson plan; armed with a body, mind, will, specific life circumstances, and an internal guidance system, we seek to discover how to use it all to find the Way 道. Ten, like one, represents unity and completion.

The seven Po

In order to make proper use of the Yi and Zhi, the disposition and orientation of the Heart-Mind in search of the Tao, we are endowed with seven lesson plans under the domain of the Po embedded within the fabric of our body-mind complex. The number seven is highly significant in the anatomy of the physical and psychic body; it is also the number of the soul and the feminine cycling of seven years. There are seven days in each phase of the menstrual cycle. The seven stars of the Big Dipper create an inner stellar framework along the midline, where we also have seven diaphragms, seven chakras, and seven major nervous plexuses. We have seven upper orifices and seven aspects of the corporeal soul, which contain the major lessons that tend to challenge us on our life journey.

The seven Po not only hold our trauma; they give rise to it. They are our greatest teachers. Until we have learned their lessons, they remain in the deep shadows of our internal landscape, waiting to be activated so they can help us progress. Programmed by Heaven at conception, they lay like dormant serpents in the underbelly, and when it is time for our lesson to emerge, predetermined life challenges will change the internal environment and wake up the Po, which, if resisted, can fester, anguishing body, mind, and soul. We can't speed them along, slow them down, jump over, or sidestep them. While we may try numerous ways to escape, medicate, or distract ourselves from them, they will come back, usually with a vengeance. Yet when we begin to recognize them, we can bow down to them as the benevolent guiding spirits that they are.

The seven Po deities (Yin, Yang, Shen, Qi, Jing, Longevity, and Sex) create the necessary friction for us to overcome on our life path. Seen as the animal souls, they are governed by the moon, and associated with the seven emotions, seven deadly sins, and seven temptations. While they are depicted as ghoulish figures with names like "Thief Swallower" and "Dead Dog," the powers of Yin usually get a bad rap. While they are not to be blindly indulged, they are not "bad," and nor are they to be avoided; they bring to life the most challenging issues that can force us out of a mundane ego-based existence to a sacred life in service to the whole. They provide the alchemical fuel that propels us all the way from the underworld to Heaven's gates, deep within our own psyche. These inner hauntings have a long history of being disowned, projected outwards, and called evil spirits. Yet when we can turn the light of consciousness around and meet them with understanding, our most demonic emotional issues turn into our greatest assets. When we go directly through the eye of the needle of our own fears, they are literally transformed into the wisdom of the lesson learned. Our constitution is cleansed.

The Po souls give rise to our baser instincts, including the desire for food, sex, and material wealth. Like hungry ghosts in their extreme forms, addictions and substance abuse belong to the Po realm. Those who need to control their intake are precisely the ones who cannot. Likewise, those who need most to undo negative or traumatic messages from their past simply cannot reach them through conscious effort. While changing negative thoughts to more positive ones might help that over which the conscious mind has control, we cannot control the unconscious. All we can do is be willing to turn toward our most challenging issues. And in order to see clearly in the dark, we need to bring the light of consciousness with us. That light is offered by the Hun.

The three Hun

The three Hun, in communication with both Heaven and the seven Po, help mediate our place between Little (individualized) Shen and Big (cosmic) Shen. They provide the intangible aspects of our higher functions: one carries the fetal spark of light; one determines the things toward which we will be attracted; and one the light of our intellect. In order to accurately utilize the Hun, they must interact with the Po. A common misunderstanding humans have made for far too long is to reject their baser instincts or suppress their most glaring issues, and "choose" the light over the darkness. This preference for Yang has made us an imbalanced, Yin-deficient species. The Hun and Po souls separate, keeping the subconscious in the dark, where much of humanity remains blind to their own inner work and live as what Zhuang Zi referred to as "walking corpses," recirculating the same putrid issues in their lives over and over. The *Ling Shu* describes in Chapter 8 a condition whereby the Hun and Po become injured, and we become mad. Because the Po's gravitational pull is in and down toward that which is unconscious, the conscious Hun must interact with them so the light of wisdom can help us navigate in the powerful darkness to learn our lessons. While it may feel maddening at times, eventually the Hun rise and the Po exit. Through this process we can become like the immortals who danced with their own darkness, trading their egos to embody the light of Shen Ming. Deeply rooted in Yin, they remain eternal beacons lighting the Way, never afraid of the dark.

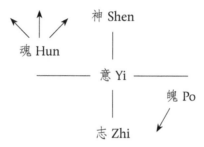

Every moment is a choice where we can pivot toward truth or ignorance. And the pivot is the center pole through which Shen, Yi, and Zhi make consciousness aware of its divinity and around which the Hun and Po souls interact, dancing their cosmic dance of evolution.

Since we come from the Tao, return to the Tao, and are Tao in between, why would Shen as Po wish to experience the sense of separation in life and all of its messiness in the first place? We might see it as the One, the collective intelligence desiring to experience manifest existence. We might attempt to explain it through a continuation of past lives, where the soul is drawn to parents who will provide the issues it needs to complete its curriculum, and call it karma. The reason, however, can only be answered by journeying through the curriculum imparted by our own souls as we discover their lessons, and discover our own destiny in this life.

Our karma, by the way, is not separate from our ancestors or our children; it forms a link throughout generations and dimensions. If we query the same of the unborn souls that may enter our lives, we will never come to a satisfactory answer. Going back to Kahlil Gibran's poem "On Children:" *Their souls dwell in the house of tomorrow, which you cannot visit, not even in your dreams.* The spirits remain mysterious and are not to be figured out. Just honored. Big Shen remains unknowable to the finite mind. The mental apparatus can only get us to a certain point, where all answers fail us. We have to come to the mystery empty of preconceived notions and surrender again and again to the wisdom of the Tao.

Curriculum

We are in this Earth School to enhance the depth and light of our souls; our curriculum, as we will see in the following pages, is implanted in utero. As we venture forth from the cosmic womb, if we choose to invest the gift of this earthly life to grow our souls rather than serve our base instincts, spirits appear to guide us on our path—without and within. Divine signposts are given along the way. As we meet and learn the curriculum set forth for us, our hardships are turned into treasures; our most troubling issues become our greatest assets. And as we courageously continue on our earthly journey, spirit is redeemed from matter like diamonds from coal. If the gift of life is spent sincerely cultivating the depth and light of our highest spiritual selves, our souls quicken in the womb of our earthly life as the coarse energies of selfishness, remorse, and greed are transformed into finer vibrations like peace, joy, and wisdom.

Finally, when our physical bodies weaken and our minds forget the mundane, we become ever-more spirit like, and can perceive the threads of Heaven that lead us home.

> Let the soul banish all that disturbs;
> let the body that envelops it be still,
> and all the frettings of the body, and all that surrounds it;
> let earth and sea and air be still, and heaven itself.
> And then let the (hu)man think of the Spirit
> as streaming, pouring, rushing and shining into him
> from all sides while (s)he stands quiet.
>
> —*Plotinus (205 AD)*

Pregnancy and renewal

So why all this talk of the soul's curriculum and life purpose when this is a book about pregnancy? Taoist teachings warn us about a time when humanity forgot to revere their souls. They lived only for themselves, warred within themselves, and became disordered. And Heaven shut its gates, depriving Earth of its light and withdrawing its vitality. There was no more surging in life, Tian Gui (the Heavenly Essence) dried up, and humanity started to perish. The humans became obsessed with reproducing their seeds, eggs, and their way of life; they tried to bypass nature and force life to conform to their desires. And Heaven waited patiently, subtly reminding them that calamity is inevitable for those who internally go against that which gives them life. Doesn't this sound eerily pertinent to where we are headed today?

Further, while Taoist teachings view the body's internal landscape as a vehicle for Jing to transform into Shen, one of the means for this metamorphosis is to treat our own body as if we are pregnant, caring for the growth of our soul as if it was an embryonic sage that we were tending to. Caring for the life of another within and caring for ourselves should not be two different things.

My decades of experience working with fertility highlighted one essential truth again and again. As much as I might have liked to help someone conceive and detour from their own curriculum, in the long run, it didn't work. While they might have been able to bypass nature and achieve pregnancies through IVF and donor gametes, I witnessed too many miscarriages, stillborns, and infants who didn't survive beyond a few earthly breaths. Life, it seems, will come out of the void when it is good and ready. Those most desperate to conceive usually come to a pivot point:

- Do they turn outward toward control, demanding Life endow them with child simply because they want it so badly? These were the ones who were rushed, stressed; they suffered the most, and were least likely to achieve success on their journey. They were simply going against nature.
- Or do they slow down, letting go of their fierce hold on how and when life was to manifest, and instead turn inward to address their own souls?

Those who followed the deeper pull and chose the latter path, perhaps against everything their rational minds were telling them, were the ones to whom Life said *yes*, often in miraculously unexpected ways. Those trying to force Heaven to conform to their wills seemed more lifeless and unreceptive, from their Hearts to the cells of their uterine linings. Perhaps Life is urging those who will be ushering in the new generation of souls during this trying time of humanity and planetary change to live by a new directive, our original one. It seems as though the universe has its own evolutionary plan, urging the life-givers to come into harmony with nature so that life can once again manifest according to the ways of Heaven.

Women from some Eastern traditions used the gestational period to overcome their own issues so they didn't pass them on to their children. The mother's state of consciousness creates the internal environment in which the fetal soul will marinate. Thus, as her soul evolves, the soul of her child becomes open for greater transformation. This is the greatest endowment we can offer our children, the gift of our own transformation so our unresolved issues don't become their legacy. Much of our discussion will utilize the ten lunar months of pregnancy, which can provide a treatment model that also applies to reconciling one with their own spirit when they have lost their way.

Fetal development is broken down into three trimesters representing the three primary themes of life—survival, interaction, and differentiation. These will become the basis of the trinity of body, mind, and soul as the three Treasures (Jing, Qi, Shen), the three Dan Tien, and the three levels of the brain and gut (hind, mid, and fore).

1. During the first trimester, the Jing is programmed by the past within the lower Dan Tien. The process is governed by Earth's ability to bank the Jing, Qi, and Blood. The cosmic life principle, the Yuan Qi, will be established by the Jing of the parents who will transmit their genetics for the Po soul to inhabit. This will establish the primary structures necessary for survival, and will define its basic constitution. If the life principle continues to be accepted, the embryo will proceed to the second, fetal stage of development.

2. Trimester two is governed by Fire and the middle Dan Tien, which rule the interactive dynamics of the soul's future life. Zong Qi, the gathering Qi of the chest, comes into play now as ancestral contributions from previous generations determine which genes will be expressed, based on epigenetic influences provided through the state of the mother. Here the soul is programmed with its upcoming curriculum that will establish its

temperament and behavioral tendencies, providing the opportunity for the soul to either establish its sovereignty or become a victim of its life circumstances.

3. The third trimester, which belongs to the upper Dan Tien, is governed by Wood, where the timeline of how the curriculum is to be carried out moment to moment will determine how the soul differentiates itself in life. Jing Shen projects, through Yintang and Baihui, experiences that will be stored and utilized to provide either new, clear vision, or become stagnant repeats of past programming.

Ten is the number of completion, attained when Hun and Po are in harmony and the Zang organs are complete. Chapter 1 of the *Su Wen* speaks of men of high antiquity who passed 100 springs and autumns because they observed the Way, modeled themselves on Yin Yang, limited activity, didn't exhaust themselves thoughtlessly, and the body and spirits held together until they departed at 100 years. Chapter 54 of the *Ling Shu* speaks of ten cycles of ten. Similarly, the development of the channel system will be intertwined within the three trimesters over ten lunar months of gestation, which we will go through in depth, but first we can make some parallels with the ten phases of a saint's life on the way to immortality, through which we are asked to renew ourselves with our soul's original contract. These aspects also follow three primary dictates: survival, interaction, and differentiation. We can always return to these phases of life where we missed some essential programming, are stuck in time through regret, or remain conflicted.

Channel	Phase of life
1 Liver	Pre-Heaven, the unseen origin on the verge of manifestation
2 Gallbladder	Infant, still undifferentiated
3 Pericardium	Child develops sense of self
4 San Jiao	Teenager or young adult, where Yin and Yang divide
5 Spleen	Identity begins to solidify
6 Stomach	Enters adulthood
7 Lung	Acquired conditioning solidifies into certain inner fixations
8 Large Intestine	Life asks us to release and let go of our inflexibility

Cont.

9 Kidney	Challenge to step up to new potential and die to the old
10 Urinary Bladder	Last choice to become mundane or celestial

Just as Chinese medicine can be used to address body, mind, and soul, pregnancy can define a physical potential where we are birthing a new being into existence; it can be used as a mythic metaphor to recover aspects of our own soul from the Mysterious Mother and lead us to awakening; or it can be both—where the souls of mother and child together honor the reasons why life chose to manifest through them in the first place. They are in this together.

Current science positions the universe as the birthing place of all entities and thus a cosmic mother. New perspectives on the birthing aspects of the universe may also help to depict the life space as one that is intended to nurture. The intricate balances of chemicals and stardust, which must occur for life to appear, mimic the process of human birth. Science provides the images of the universe as initiating or siring and as an expanding womb, ready to sustain life. The birthing is mathematical, complex, and necessary. We are made in the image of a parent or creator who invites us into a cosmic belonging... "We need the embrace of a Cosmic Mother" (Barbara A. Holmes, Race and the Cosmos).

CHAPTER 2

Dynamics of the Creation Process

The valley spirit never dies;
it is called the Mysterious Feminine.
The doorway of the Mysterious Feminine
is the root of heaven and earth.
Continuous, on the brink of existence
like a gossamer veil, barely seen.
Use it as you will.
It will never run dry.

—Tao Te Ching (Book of the Way), Chapter 6

Life emerges from the spirit of the valley. Hidden from view, we are recipients of creation. While nature doesn't flaunt or openly reveal her secrets, we can peer into the mystery through various lenses. Here we will venture into the dynamics of creation using various reproductive models to explain how the macrocosm becomes the microcosm, blending biomedical systems, structural anatomy, the ancient Chinese understanding of natural cycles, and myths to develop an understanding of fertility. Without losing the sense of the miraculous, let's look at some of the systems life uses to wrap itself into being.

Ovarian biorhythms behind the scene

Fourteenth century mystic Lalla likened the soul to the moon, *new, and always new again*, and to the continuously creating ocean. She invites us to scour our mind and body until we too are new each moment until, like Lalla, we *Live in the soul...* until we begin to go naked and dance (Naked Song, Coleman Barks, Pilgrim Publishing, 2006). One night per year, in sync with the correct water temperatures and the shining of a particular full moon, entire colonies of coral reefs, responding to precise lunar cues, simultaneously release blizzards of eggs and sperm into the depths of the ocean floor. Nature, continually creating, replenishes life, teeming forth with possibility. Because the body is a microcosm of nature, we, too, are new, each moment new, continuously creating.

During fetal development, we are endowed with a primordial pool of follicles that number about a million at birth, half that many at menarche, and continuing to about 10,000 as we enter into the perimenopausal years. These primordial follicles, which have been present since we were fetuses in our mother's womb, remain unchanged, pure potential until they start interacting with our internal environment. Let's stop there and take in this important bit of information. They persist in a protected, unaffected state—the same as when we were three-and-a-half and fourteen. So what happens when we reach our forties and we're told our eggs are old? Well, immutable as the primordial follicles remain, when they start interacting with our Qi and Blood, they begin to morph into a reflection of how nature reads our internal cues. Our eggs, held within an electromagnetic field of potential, don't actually undergo the effects of aging until they come into contact with the potentially degenerating effects of how we utilize our Jing and what we are financing with our Qi and Blood.

Up to a year before ovulation, from deep within the ovary a push of Yuan Qi releases tiny follicles to leave their primordial pool and enter into the growing assembly of follicles that begin to move through various phases of development on their march toward ovulation. Yuan Qi is dense, slow, and contains the information provided by nature and our ancestry. Belonging to the collective and operating below the level of consciousness, Yuan Qi ensures the continuation of the species, but is indifferent to our personal desires. The initial impulse is driven by the strength of the Yuan Qi, the internal force that will propel them forward until one of them is selected for ovulation. Each egg gets one attempt to reach the finish line. The unselected follicles will go into atresia, their final resting place, never to be revived again. An inside determinant will select one follicle and prime its cells to respond to small amounts of follicle-stimulating hormone (FSH), a Yang hormone released by the pituitary gland. The chosen one is known as the dominant follicle that will grow to about the size of a large grape before it releases the mature egg it has been coddling and caring for since fetal life, which has been eavesdropping on its host's physical, mental, and emotional states for about a year now, mimicking her every move.

About three months prior to ovulation and thirteen lunar months or one calendar year prior to birth, folliculogenesis begins as the follicles enter the all important tonic growth phase where protein synthesis occurs. Inside the follicle, the egg is bathed in clear Jin fluid, which will provide the environmental cues it needs to know what type of external environment it will have to survive in if it is to become a human being. This is where it becomes informed by Ying or nutritive Qi, which is now influenced by our nutritional state, circulatory and oxygenation capacity, life interactions, emotional states, and conscious desires. Right here, consciousness through a new electromagnetic field is already actively choosing its expression and lining up those chromosomes to go along with what is perceived—physically, mentally, and emotionally. Conscious and unconscious stressors—all is taken in—lead to genetic instability. As the macrocosm is captured by the soul it embodies, the germ cells apprehend the microcosm by lining up the genetic code to meet it.

As we go through our day, our body-minds are constantly making unconscious micro adjustments to blood flow and hormonal output, as well as millions of other survival functions. The hypothalamus, the master gland of all endocrine and therefore reproductive functions, picks up these internal cues and translates them into hormone-stimulating factors based upon our emotional response to our environment. If our environment is perceived through a stressful or threatening lens, our nutritive Qi will carry threatening types of chemicals. Our blood will tend to be more acidic. Our stress hormones will dominate the reproductive hormones, and the follicular fluid in which the eggs are developing will be more stagnant and asphyxiating. Oxidative stress will dominate, choking out growth-enhancing proteins and hormones. And the egg will receive the message to morph its chromosomes into a genetic equation that might possibly survive in this stressful environment. Chinese medical patterns include Qi stagnation, Dampness, Heat, or Blood stasis on a background of Qi and Blood deficiency. The result: poor egg quality, which will become poor embryo quality, often inconsistent with life. Or we perceive the world and ourselves in all of our flawed magnificence; we still try to honor the cycles in nature, break toxic patterns, eat right, rest well, and open up to all of the beauty in life. The result: stronger Jing and brighter Shen, which the Qi and Blood follow. Regardless of maternal age, this is the recipe for quality eggs.

Preconception preparation begins well before deciding to mix egg and sperm together. And a major focus that will determine the physical, mental, and emotional health of the child it is capable of becoming is to start lightening the external and internal loads on our health and wellbeing. The time to reduce stress and live as if new life is being carried within is always now.

The Essence and its container: Tian Gui and Zi Gong

Uterine Blood is full of the purest vital Essences capable of producing life. Tian Gui describes the spilling forth of the Heavenly Essence that is required to initiate the impulse for life. After two cycles of seven (although now it is more like two cycles of five-and-a-half), when a girl has been supplied with sufficient Essence to propel her from childhood into womanhood, she is given the gift of being able to support the life of another. Arising from the internal depths, in fact the very Yin of Yin, an unseen force spills forth from Heaven to infuse her being, connecting her to the moon and her lunar cycles. This heavenly libation is poured forth as a superabundance of Essences containing the natural authenticity of life. When this Heavenly Essence bubbles forth, it trickles down from the celestial streams in the center of the brain into the life-giving powers of the Heart, whose Fire now calls up the Water from the Kidneys to sync with the phases of the moon. The precious life-giving Blood, Tian Gui, is the result.

The Uterus is considered one of the Curious Organs, which, along with the Brain, Gallbladder, Mai, Marrow, and Bones, are the evolutionary systems responsible for survival and perpetuation of the species. While Zang Fu generally remain the same, Curious Organs mutate to orient and adapt to changing environments. We are in changing times and cycles are speeding up. Yuan Qi, the unfolding of our constitutional energetics, can barely keep up with the expediting cycles of seven when the body has a chance to rewire itself. So, when we speak of the womb, we are not speaking merely of a fleshy muscular organ in the lower burner; we are speaking about the potential space that houses the most prized process by which regeneration takes place.

The mother is the conduit through which humans evolve, and she had better keep up or the Yuan Qi, indifferent to her personal desires, may try to mutate on its own, and you know where that leaves us—with chromosomal combinations incompatible with life. Now that doesn't mean that she is to rev herself up to keep with the changing environment; quite the opposite, in fact. She is to slow down, go within, and recover the natural cyclic rhythm Heaven has imprinted within her.

As the Heart has endowed the womb with the remarkable ability to bring forth life, it needs an equally exceptional container: one that can hold the most precious seedling of life and intimately grow it into a human being. Zi Gong (Palace of the Child) includes the ovary, fallopian tube, uterus, and cervix, which together comprise the Curious Organ that will house the fetus while it is suspended between Heaven and Earth. Bao Mai refers to the Jing–Shen relationship between the uterus and Heart, and Bao Luo links the Kidneys with the womb. Du 1 Pomen (Long Strong) and Ren 15 Jiuwei (Turtledove Tail), form the source Luo connection that the vertical Bao Mai and horizontal Bao Luo will follow as they weave together the Conception, Governing, Penetrating, and Belt meridians to secure the child as it ascends toward Ren 14 Juque (Great Palace Gateway). During the ninth month of pregnancy, this network of communication will begin to separate.

The Bao 包 is the primal wrapping that envelops the origin of life—ours or another's. Its character is comprised of a fetus spiraling 巳 counterclockwise according to pre-Heaven's reverse cycle, wrapped in the embrace of a womb 勹 that spirals clockwise, like post-Heaven's Sheng cycle. Form and formlessness dance together in the dark womb, where spirit takes form. Attached to Ming Men, Bao is connected to the Zang Fu, Qi, and Blood of the mother as this sacred spiral embodies the most efficient geometric form in nature through which becoming and returning proceed. Pre-Heaven embraces post-Heaven as the soul spirals from its cosmic origin into its earthly domain.

Just as Bao 包 is the primal wrapping of the embryo, Bao 抱 also refers to an embrace. The first embrace is the acceptance of embodiment, a function of the Conception Vessel. At the moment of conception the spirit has the purpose of her life whispered into her ear as she passes the heavenly gateway into life. It may sound something like this:

> You are passing into the realm of earthly aliveness. The primary requirement will
> be to receive nourishment in order to find your true self. If you accept, you'll be

challenged to find your deepest inner resources to carry out this responsibility of living life in a balanced way. You will never, ever be abandoned, although at times you may feel forsaken. You are only borrowed here; at any time, you may return.

The *Bao Pu Zi* 抱樸子 was a Taoist text written by the alchemist and Jin dynasty scholar Ge Hong (283–343 CE), who was known as Bao Pu Zi, the one who embraces simplicity. This refers to returning to the desireless state of the sage who is united with the Tao, like an infant. We can accept life fully, we can return to the Tao while we are very much alive, and we can leave earthly existence and return to the origin any time along the journey. When a fetus returns to the Tao (miscarries) in utero, from this side of the veil, it may seem like a grave mistake. But from the eyes of the Spirit of All That Is, it's all good. The way of the Tao is to return. Tao is there at the beginning, at the end, and everywhere in between. The Tao does not err.

Two cycles—forward and reverse generative cycles

The *Tao Te Ching (Book of the Way)* tells us that the Tao remains unborn yet becomes all things. But first the One must become the Two. Between nonexistence and existence are two interactive dynamics, one pre-heavenly and one post-heavenly, that create life. While we never forget the one energy that rides between them, let's look at their interplay.

First there is the unseen, unborn substratum of counterentropic energy operating below our awareness. Yet as we have seen, we can access this universal energy at any time. It has never been born and thus can never die. The *Tao Te Ching (Book of the Way)* refers to this power as the Valley Spirit. Chinese medicine calls it prenatal. This power operates via the reverse generative (Sheng) cycle, where Fire returns to Wood and Wood returns to Water. While life longs to express itself, it is countered by an opposing urge to return to its origin to be nurtured by the Mysterious Mother. The reverse creation cycle governs menstruation, where Heaven endlessly cycles backwards and pours itself into Earth to create the stuff of life. Tian Gui and the gynecological cycle are under reverse cycle dominance.

The process begins with Metal, as all new endeavors are preceded by relinquishing the old. Metal, which represents form, governs the release of menstrual blood, as the Lungs direct the Qi to begin a new cycle. In the same way a finger placed on the top of a straw will uphold water inside, the Lung dynamic (Lu 7 Lieque (Broken Sequence) opens the Conception Vessel) allows the Da Bao energies of the chest to descend to the pelvic basin and release that which the Dai Mai has held. Then Earth, which provides shape, takes over, as the dynamics of the Spleen and Stomach produce the Blood of the upcoming cycle (Sp 4 Gongsun (Grandfather-Grandson), Sp 6 Sanyinjiao (Three Yin Intersection)). The Spleen must then be able to ascend to the Heart (Ki 2 Rangu (Blazing Valley), Sp 8 Diji (Earth Pivot), St 36 Zusanli (Leg Three Miles)). The Heart will then charge the Blood with the fiery redness of spirit (Ren 14 Juque (Great Palace Gateway), Ren 17 Tanzhong (Center Temple)), which the Pericardium must cool (Pc 8 Laogong (Labor Palace)) before it is sent to the Liver. Wood represents the universal creative urge, and the Liver, which holds the nourishing Blood (Lv 3 Taichong (Great Surge), Lv 8 Ququan (Spring at the Bend)), will be responsible for doling it out to the Kidneys (Ki 3 Taixi (Supreme Stream), UB 23 Shenshu (Kidney Transporter)). The Tao is like Water, which holds our oceanic potential, and the Kidney will oversee the development of the uterine lining through the Bao Lou, the connection between the Kidneys and the womb (Zi Gong).

The pre-heavenly reverse cycle will govern the soul's incarnation through gestation as Water provides the Jing through which Metal Po will be earthed into this enfleshed existence; Fire will impart the curriculum and Wood will provide the impetuous finale of birth.

The pre-heavenly origin gives rise to the post-heavenly manifest expression of things like buds in the springtime and new babies that belong to the generative cycle, where Water nourishes Wood, Wood engenders Fire, etc. While the reverse cycle governs the gynecological system, the forward cycle regulates hormones and thus the endocrine system. Our daily interactive consciousness lives primarily in this realm of space-time where the sun rises and sets, and our constitution is shaped by life circumstances that give rise to how the postnatal Qi of the twelve regular meridians will flow. This is the realm of entropy—because things are being generated, they are also declining. Babies become children, adults, elderly, and return to the Tao. The endocrine system governs and constantly attempts to harmonize this dynamic to maintain equilibrium through the ever-fluctuating changes in life. In this cycle, Water produces Wood during the follicular phase; Fire governs ovulation; Earth sustains the luteal phase; and Metal releases to begin the cycle again.

The generative cycle perpetuates; the reverse cycle rebirths and renews.

Together one cycles forward, one backward, just like a live infinity symbol moving in both directions, both necessary for the continuation of life. The left, prenatal side moves counterclockwise through the first ancestry (Conception, Governing and prenatal Penetrating Meridian) of the Eight Extraordinary Meridians, all conduits of prenatal Source Qi. The right, postnatal flows clockwise into the Sheng cycle, which governs the Zang Fu. They rely on and nourish one another through the bridge between the postnatal Penetrating Meridian or Chong Mai. The first ancestry is conditioned and socialized into the shape and function of second and third ancestries, which consist of the Wei (network), Qiao (heel), and Dai (belt) vessels of the Eight Extraordinary Meridians. The ancestry model isn't fixed; it describes relationships. For the purposes of conception, the Penetrating Meridian brings them all together—linking up pre- and postnatal energies and bridging the Eight Extraordinary Meridians with the Zang Fu.

The moon rises and sets within

The phases of the menstrual cycle harmonize the mother with the tides of nature. The earliest treatments for irregular menstrual cycles advised women to sleep outside in nature for one lunar cycle to sync with the cycles of the moon. Women of old also practiced moon gazing to absorb the power of lunar light, especially during a full moon.

Outer lunar cycles

Lunar cycles, described in Chapter 26 of the *Su Wen*, influence menstrual rhythms. The Moon is seen to gather water, and Earth absorbs vital essence from the Moon. We can absorb this cosmic Essence through the bottom of the feet at Ki 1 Yongquan (Bubbling Spring), and we can gaze at the Moon to absorb its Essence through our eyes. During a full moon, the Qi and Blood are full, and Yang Qi travels to the sinews where Qi and Blood converge. The muscles become strong; hence we are advised not to tonify during the full moon, and should avoid needling command points like Ll 4 Hegu (Joining Valley) and convergent points of the Yang sinews (SI 18 Quanliao (Cheek Bone Crevice), St 3 Juliao (Great Crevice), St 8 Touwei (Head Corner), GB 13 Benshen (Root Spirit)) during the full moon. However, if Qi and Blood are deficient, we can needle the convergent points of the Yin sinews (Ren 3 Zhongji (Central Pole), GB 22 Yuanye (Armpit

Abyss)) during the full moon to divert Blood into the ancestral sinews. In the same regard, we are advised not to sedate during the new moon, when Qi and Blood are effectively empty, and when needling can further reduce Wei Qi.

Lunar and menstrual phases

The new moon corresponds to menses—a time of rest and inner quiet to reflect on new beginnings. Treatment strategies move Liver Qi and Heart Blood, and help the Lungs to release.

The first quarter represents the follicular phase of fresh growth and creative inspiration. Nourish Kidney Yin, Liver Blood, and Spleen Qi.

The full moon equates with the ovulatory cycle where energies are high; because this is also a time of opening, exercise discernment. Move the Qi, Quicken the Blood, and nourish the Spleen.

The last quarter represents the luteal phase where we are in a holding pattern—evaluating where we have been, finishing up what we have started, and being open to begin again. Regulate Liver Blood and Qi, tonify and warm Kidneys.

Inner lunar cycles

The dark moon begins a new cycle at Zi Gong and will wax its way up the Chong Mai (Penetrating Vessel) throughout each menstrual cycle. Remember the Chong Mai contains a great power through which the heaviness of Earth can be raised if we walk our life correctly; ever becoming lighter as the seed of potential is animated with the vigor of the ascending movement of life up this very efficient route of communication; filling up the Sea of Blood. The energies of the rising crescent moon will emerge at Ki 11 Henggu (Pubic Bone) and ascend up the first trajectory of the Chong Mai to Ki 21 Youmen (Hidden Gate) (where the fetus will peak after its ten lunar months in utero). As the lunar energies rise up the front, they lift through the upper Kidney spirit points, passing Ki 27 Shufu (Shu Mansion) and lift to Ren 24 Chengjiang (Receiving Fluid), where the tongue connects via the upper palate to the Du Mai (Governing Vessel), as the full moon reaches the celestial peaks at Du 20 Baihui (Hundred Convergences). As the full moon shines above, down below the ovule is ripening to the surface of the follicle, and the lower regions become more and more Yin. The cervix softens and lifts toward the center of the body as it flowers open to allow passage of sperm. As Yin reaches its apogee, the moon shines on Yintang, releasing celestial dew as luteinizing hormone (LH) showers forth from the pituitary gland. The ovule is discharged. The follicle becomes a yellow corpus luteum, like the embryo's Spleen, which will shower forth the hormones it will need to survive. The moon begins to wane.

Meanwhile, as the Chong Mai governs ascent up the front, a complementary descending process occurs. Like a weighted pulley down the back, Wei Qi simultaneously descends down the Du Mai at the rate of one vertebra each of the 28 days, according to the *Ling Shu*. Beginning at Du 17 Naohu (Brain's Door), the new cycle begins, and the Qi will descend one vertebral process per day, reaching Du 10 Lingtai (Soul's Tower) (which addresses mental obstacles to ascending our present peak or Heart pain) around ovulation. (You can palpate the space below the corresponding spinous processes to see if any areas are flaccid or gummy; if so, needle them so the Qi can pass through freely.) As Yin is peaking below, Qi moves inward, ensuring only sperm will be allowed in, and not seminal fluid.

If egg and sperm embrace in the Mysterious Pass, Yin and Yang will continue to interpenetrate as cellular division proceeds, rolling the compact ball of activated Jing into two and four and eight cells, into a morula and finally a blastocyst. As it makes its passage through the fallopian tube, the little ball of life will be carried along by millions of delicate cilia that will usher its arrival in the uterine cavity to make its entrance on about day 21. Yet the palace must be properly prepared. The Wei Qi must halt its descent and instead herald the opening of life's passage at Du 4 Mingmen (Gate of Destiny), where the Ministerial Fire shifts to enter the Chong Mai to allow the mingling of Heart Fire and Kidney Water in the warm hearth of Zi Gong.

By now this somewhat foreign invader (not self, but also not non-self) will be attempting to burrow into the uterine lining in order to share in the mother's blood supply. The Wei Qi has to do some fancy T cell maneuvering to block the embryo from immune attack, a pattern that involves softening the Liver, and lifting and harmonizing the Qi while ensuring the Blood flows freely.

The moon won't go down on this new being in the making; it will cycle ten times within until it is ready for birthing. If there is no spark of life, the Wei Qi will descend down the rest of the spinal column to Du 2 Yaoshu (Lumber Shu), where, with the Lung's help, the uterine Blood will be released, and the cycle will begin again.

Menstrual cycle functioning and emotional correlations

The primary job of Chinese gynecologists is to regulate menstruation. If the cycles are irregular, harmonize the Qi. If they are too short or too long, tonify the deficient energy and resolve whatever excess is present. If menstruation is excessive, tonify Qi, invigorate Blood, or clear Heat. Make sure the uterine Blood is flowing smoothly; that the Kidneys are consolidating; the Spleen is producing Blood; the Heart enlivening it; the Pericardium is cooling it; the Liver holding it; and the Lung releasing it.

Menstrual cycles can give us a clear idea about how one is living their life and the effect of any unresolved emotional factors lurking within. Li Dong Yuan's concept of Yin Fire included the idea that emotional suppression will consume the Essence, and lead to empty Heat. Zhu Dan Xi furthered the idea of depressed emotional causes of disease. Sun Si Miao stated in the *Bie Fang*,

> Women's disorders are ten times more difficult to treat than men's... Women's cravings and desires exceed men's, and they contract illness at twice the rate of men. In addition, they are imbued with affection and passion, love and hatred, envy and jealousy, and worry and rancor, which are lodged firmly in them. Since they are unable to control their emotions by themselves, the roots of their disorders are deep, and it is difficult to obtain a cure in their treatment.

> —*Sabine Wilms' translation from Nurturing the Foetus in Medieval China*

Most of us would take offense to this Yin insult (as well as his advice to pull her hair, splash vinegar in her face, and drink her husband's urine) while simultaneously admitting that some of it is true, albeit misunderstood. Women do seem to be imbued with more emotional complexity. Yet this is our superpower. Before men were in rule, families were run by the matriarch, and the goddesses wielded the power. They didn't "control" their passionate intensity; their unbridled power brought about dramatic results. In order for our treatments to reach beyond the *deep roots of our disorders* and obtain a cure, we must understand the energetic physiology of our unique emotional makeup and its cyclical nature. Then we can use our feeling power without letting it rule us.

One of the ways we harmonize with our environment is through our emotional response. When we're afraid, the Qi descends. When angry, Qi ascends. Worry knots the Qi, joy scatters the Qi, and sadness makes the Qi disappear.

Since Qi directs the Blood and Blood follows the Qi, this will obviously impact the flow of menses. Emotional extremes, which also include recirculating emotions and emotional suppression, can deplete the Qi, and cause it to stagnate. Any emotional excess can injure its Zang organ; and each in turn can agitate the Heart. When emotional imbalances arise, the pulse will lose the proper tension of its wave. It may be weak, tight, choppy, or scattered.

At the end of each menstrual cycle, if there is no pregnancy, there is an inner loss. Demise of the corpus luteum lowers estradiol and progesterone levels, which provide the negative feedback the hypothalamus and pituitary gland need to increase FSH to recruit new follicles to grow for the next cycle. New hope always begins with releasing the old. Blood and Qi fall. Because the Blood contains our emotions, we begin by feeling them and letting them go so the Heart can return to rest.

Western medicine considers the hypothalamus the control center by which the endocrine system acclimates to our environment, setting up the release of pulsatile factors that will govern menstruation. Deep in the center of the brain, invisible sensory antennae pick up signals from within and without; these signals are emotionally interpreted and converted into currents of Qi. The entire endocrine symphony begins behind the nose, an area governed by the organizing principle of Metal (Lung and Large Intestine). Primitive nose cells in the developing embryo secrete gonadotropic-releasing hormone (GnRH), which then migrate to their final destination at the base of the brain at the intersection between the nervous and endocrine systems, the junction of pain and pleasure. This function will regulate endocrine functions to harmonize with our environment for life. Just like the *Su Wen* tells us in Chapter 8, Heaven and Earth come together through the breath.

We acclimate to our environment primarily by light, smell, and temperature. The Lung, which governs the left cerebral hemisphere, and the Liver, which governs the right, mark the passage of time—past and future—and between them, the empty center, always at rest, allows the light of Heaven to shine into the darkness. Like the Earth element, the hypothalamus occupies a center role where impulses come together. This could be associated with Huang Ting Jing—the Yellow Inner Court, referring to the imperial castle's sacred center, where the Emperor and his ministers would come together to discover and carry out the will of Heaven throughout the kingdom. This is precisely what the hypothalamus does in the center of the brain to rule our inner queendom.

The hypothalamus controls, among many other functions, the regulation of the monthly ovulatory cycle, releasing thyrotrophin, corticotrophin, gonadotropin, growth hormone-releasing hormones, somatostatin, and dopamine. The pulsatile release of GnRH depends upon a number of factors:

- rhythmic signals from the environment including light-dark signals from the pineal gland, eating, sleeping, waking, working, exercising, relating (with others)
- psychological interpretation of our environment through the limbic system
- negative feedback from the gonadal hormones.

The hypothalamic Qi impulses will then be translated by the pituitary gland into regulatory hormones, setting off the cascade of thick fluids coursing through the waterways. While almost all emotional and lifestyle factors impact hypothalamic functioning, and all points on the body can feed back to impact the hypothalamus, direct points are located at Du 16 Fengfu (Wind Mansion), Du 17 Naohu (Brain's Door), and UB 10 Tianzhu (Celestial Pillar). Hypothalamic dysfunction is primarily addressed through the Eight Extraordinary Meridians. The Conception and Governing Meridians link at the hypothalamic pituitary junction at Yintang and their corresponding Yin and Yang Heel Vessels meet at UB 1 Jingming (Bright Eyes). Our initial bonding and nurturing energies come together with how we see ourselves in this moment, establishing the basic Conception and Yin Heel Vessel functioning as Lu 7 Lieque (Broken Sequence) links with Ki 6 Zhaohai (Shining Sea). The Governing Vessel carries the initial impulses of interest and curiosity in the world. Its opening point, SI 3 Houxi (Back Stream), links with Yang Heel Vessel at UB 62 Shenmai (Extending Vessel), which interfaces with the outer world, establishing our actions, protections, and defenses.

Menstrual cycle phases
Menses
Menstruation is all about releasing. Lung Qi moves the Heart Blood, which descends to the uterus via Bao Mai. The Heart–Kidney communication can be obstructed by any counterflow Qi, or Qi obstruction in the middle Dan Tien. Unacknowledged depression, grief, or loss can disrupt the menstrual cycle.

This does not mean we shouldn't experience those emotions, but that we don't suppress or overindulge in them. The *Jia Yi Jing* says that when the Lung is full of grief, its lobes become elevated and the cardiac ligation becomes tense. A common pattern experienced by those trying to conceive with the onset of each period is the refusal to acknowledge the sadness from the loss of a hoped-for thing. Instead, they put on a "positive" face and tell themselves that next cycle will be better, while the Heart longs to release the tears and fall apart a little bit. What's worse is when their practitioner cheers them on instead of acknowledging the depth of sorrow lurking beneath the smile, empty of Shen. When the Qi of the chest isn't allowed to empty, this can impact Heart Yin, which may lead to empty Fire, causing early menstruation or spotting due to Heat.

Blood stasis is another common pattern that impacts the flow of Tian Gui, perhaps causing severe menstrual pain. Sometimes the underlying pattern is that there is no inlet or outlet for the life force moving through the Heart–Kidney axis, which hinders the ability to flow. Uterine and Heart Blood stasis results, which can manifest as lack of the inherent joy of being, which the Heart provides. Ecstasy has been defined as the state where there is no stasis. In fact, the word "ecstasy" was originally used by 17th-century mystical writers to describe a rapturous state when the soul could stand outside one's self to contemplate divine states of consciousness. And yet we can't be released from our own bondage until we have gone through the things that obstruct the Heart. When we acknowledge some of our unseen beliefs, we can release them and move on.

When stuck emotions obstruct proper menstrual flow, consider releasing the Da Bao. Points like GB 22 Yuanye (Armpit Abyss), Ren 17 Tanzhong (Center Temple), Ren 14 Juque (Great Palace Gateway), Pc 6 Neiguan (Inner Pass), and Ki 21–27 can be used in conjunction with points like Sp 6 Sanyinjiao (Three Yin Intersection), Sp 8 Diji (Earth Pivot), Lv 5 Ligou (Woodworm Canal), Lv 6 Zhongdu, and Lv 8 Ququan (Spring at the Bend) that regulate the lower burner and move uterine Blood. Lu 4 Xiabai moves Lung Qi to move Heart Blood, and Lu 7 Lieque (Broken Sequence) opens the Conception Vessel. While Tian Wang Bu Xin Dan (Heavenly Empress' Special Pill to Tonify the Heart) harmonizes the Heart and Kidneys, we may need formulae that are more invigorating of the Heart and/or Uterus. Combining the ideas of Dan Shen Yin (Salvia Decoction) or Xue Fu Zhu Yu Tang (Drive Out Stasis in the Mansion of Blood Decoction) to move the Heart Blood along with formulae to move uterine Blood such as Gui Zhi Fu Ling Wan (Cinnamon Twig and Poria Pill) or Wen Jing Tan (Warm the

Menses Decoction) can address both. Shao Fu Zhu Yu Tang (Drive Out Blood Stasis in the Lower Abdomen Decoction) may be appropriate when pain is due to uterine Blood stasis.

Ovarian follicular phase or endometrial proliferative phase

This is the phase of new growth and new possibility. As the follicle grows, the uterine lining grows and proliferates, thickening itself for possible implantation. The dominant follicle whose cells have been primed to respond to small amounts of FSH releases estradiol, which promotes growth and makes us feel good—hopeful, in fact. But hope can be a nebulous and dangerous thing if we don't understand its energy. It is not the same as expecting our desires to be fulfilled. Hope is a natural buoyancy, alive in this moment, which is not tied to future outcomes. To put it simply—the Heart is filled with hope when the spirits are present. And the spirits are present now. Hope is kept alive by keeping the light of awareness within. Ht 7 Shenmen (Spirit Gate) has been found to moderate dopamine, the desire neurotransmitter, and raise neuropeptide Y in the amygdala, decreasing the fight or flight response.

Two cycles are simultaneously going on:

1. Generative (Sheng) cycle: Kidney Yin engenders Liver Blood to build the uterine lining. Kidney Yin holds our most basic substance—Jing—our very sense of being ourselves. When our sense of self is lacking—not in the egoic sense, but when we just feel an underlying insubstantiality or insecurity about who we are—all other Yin and Blood functions that rely on the Kidneys will be insufficient. Yin deficiency can also result when we refuse to accept what is. When desires exceed Liver Blood's capacity to attain the hoped-for thing, lack of hope and despondency (which stifles the Qi) result; this can lengthen the follicular phase. The Liver, which loves orderly reaching, can only reach as far as the lubrication of Liver Blood allows, or forced movement tends to produce stagnation and Heat. Make sure the Kidneys are supplemented (Ki 3 Taixi (Supreme Stream), Ki 6 Zhaohai (Shining Sea), Ki 7 Fuliu (Returning Current), UB 23 Shenshu (Kidney Transporter), UB 52 Zhishi (Will Chamber); Liu Wei Di Huang Wan (Six Ingredient Pill with Rehmannia) or Er Zhi Wan (Two Ultimate Pill)) and Liver Blood is adequate (Sp 4 Gongsun (Grandfather-Grandson), Lv 8 Ququan (Spring at the Bend), Dang Gui Shao Yao San (Angelica and

Peony Powder)). When Yin and Blood are deficient, Liver and Heart Fire may result, which can lead to frenetic activity that disrupts the Heart–Kidney axis and shortens the follicular phase. Restoring their connection may involve Tian Wang Bu Xin Dang (Heavenly Empress' Pill to Tonify the Heart), using the first and second trajectories of Chong Mai (Sp 4 Gongsun (Grandfather-Grandson)), and choosing points from Ki 11–27 based on palpation.

2. During the reverse generative cycle, the Spleen is building Blood and lifting it to the Heart. It is imperative that the Spleen not be bogged down by overthinking or worry. Impaired Spleen function can lead to Dampness, which can then drain into the lower burner putting out the Ming Men Fire. Failure of Spleen Qi to ascend to the Heart can also result in Spleen and Blood deficiency. Gui Pi Tang (Restoring the Spleen Decoction) will be more useful when Heart Blood is deficient, while Bu Zhong Yi Qi Tang (Tonify the Middle and Augment the Qi Decoction) will lift sunken Qi. Consider St 36 Zusanli (Leg Three Miles), Sp 4 Gongsun (Grandfather-Grandson), Sp 6 Sanyinjiao (Three Yin Intersection), UB 20 Pishu (Spleen's Hollow), and Du 20 Baihui (Hundred Convergences).

Whenever we are in the initial pursuit to fulfill a longing, we are advised to keep it within rather than exhaust our Qi and Blood trying to reach without. The Shen of the Heart literally can't reach the Kidney Essence if the desire pulls one too strongly outside. This depletes Kidney Yin, which makes the body want to hold on to Yin in the form of estradiol E2. Because E2 is a growth hormone, when the body tries to retain it, pathological growths can result in the form of Dampness and Qi stagnation. Ovarian cysts, tumorous growths, and cancers may result. Here we must simultaneously nourish the self (Kidneys), and provide invigorating movement (joy and hope) in life. Thus, we have to, at least temporarily, get out of the external desire business.

So how do we do this without causing more stagnation from denying our emotional wanting? We hold the feeling in our Heart of what we want most, and begin to live it. If what you want most is to experience the sense of loving or being loved, imagine it, feel it in your heart, let it course through your system, and start to live from its fullness rather than its lack. We must love our lives as they are before we pretend that we will get satisfaction from what we do not have.

Ovulation

Ovulation is a very dynamic time that belongs to the Heart. Chapter 66 of the *Su Wen* says that when a substance reaches its limit, it is said to be changed. Yin, in the form of estrogen, has peaked, which now triggers the release of LH to release the egg below. Liver Blood engenders Heart Qi in the forward cycle; Heart Blood offers itself to the Liver in the reverse cycle. The cervix, fallopian tube, and the Heart all flower into an open state during ovulation, at which time the Wei Qi increases and moves inward to keep out any pathogenic factors. Because of all this activity in the Heart, there may be a rise in felt emotions, so it's important to keep the Heart moving and light. It is crucial to address any limitation in the expression of who we are. Feeling oppressed, suppressed, or depressed by life circumstances can stagnate the Qi, and close off the Heart. Remedy this by opening the thoracic cavity. Teach your patients to use their diaphragms to breathe fully into the lower Dan Tien. In the meantime, Gua Sha around the diaphragm can resolve stagnant Qi and Blood that might have collected in the chest or breast area. The Pericardium must cool the Heart Blood before sending it to the Liver, so Pc 8 Laogong (Labor Palace) or Dan Shen Yin (Salvia Decoction) might be appropriate during this time; discontinue if conception is confirmed through the pulse or positive pregnancy test.

Ovarian luteal phase or endometrial secretory phase

After Yin has reached its peak, and the follicle has discharged its ovule, the corpus luteum produces the dominant hormone of the luteal phase, progesterone, which produces a feeling that everything is going to be okay. The generative cycle moves from the Heart to the Spleen, whose Qi must lift and hold, with support from Kidney Yang. Worry, anxiety, and overthinking hinder the Spleen's ability to hold things like embryos and emotions in their proper place. When the Spleen is taxed by worry, Dampness can be the result, which lack of movement only worsens. The luteal phase, contrary to popular belief, is the time to move the Qi, not to sit around, fearful that one might or might not be pregnant. Keep the Qi moving with relaxed and moderate exercise. Kidney Yang is necessary for consolidating and grasping the Qi, which fear will inhibit. Express worry and fear to release them; don't suppress. UB 20 Pishu (Spleen's Hollow), UB 23 Shenshu (Kidney Transporter), Bu Zhong Yi Qi Tang (Tonify the Middle and Augment the Qi Decoction), Si Jun Zi Tang (Four Gentlemen Decoction), and Jin Gui Shen Qi Wan (Kidney Qi Pill from the Golden Cabinet) might be appropriate formulas.

Because the reverse generative cycle requires that the Liver Blood go to the Kidney Yin to support the uterine lining, it is important to nourish Liver Blood and regulate Liver Qi, especially as we move closer to the premenstrum. Emotional resistance to life, frustration, and anger (all on a continuum of the same energy—*I want things to be different than they are*) blocks the Liver's ability to nourish Kidney Essence.

Implantation can be enhanced with Lv 8 Ququan (Spring at the Bend) and Pc 7 Daling (Great Mound), and herbs that nourish Liver Blood such as Bai Shao (white peony) and Dang Gui (angelica). Dang Gui Shao Yao San (Angelica and Peony Powder), Xiao Yao San (Free and Easy Wanderer Powder), or Dan Zhi Xiao Yao San (Bupleurum and Peony Formula) with additions may be appropriate. While Chong Wei Zi (leonurus fruit) and Yi Mu Cao (Chinese motherwort) are typically contraindicated during pregnancy, they can help build and move endometrial Blood during the secretory phase.

Qi and Blood are high in preparation for life, and can produce some symptoms of excess if there is no new life to support. If there is no conception, the Lungs will redirect the process by signaling the corpus luteum to cease progesterone production. Levels fall, the uterine lining liquifies, and like a finger taken off the top of a straw, the Blood is released. A new cycle begins.

The two cycles circulate forward and backward between Heaven and Earth like an infinity symbol; while the forward Sheng cycle governs our basic response to life circumstances, we need the reverse cycle energetic to create new possibilities. Prenatal creation must include the study of embryology. Water is our starting place, where we recognize who and what is being recreated, and includes the sexual energy of parents. Metal calls in the Celestial Qi from the Universe. Earth provides the foundational fleshy substance; Heart provides movement; and Wood initiates new processes into being.

Commonly used herbal fertility formulae
Follicular phase strategies
Tonify Qi, Blood, and Yin; resolve any stasis, Dampness, or stagnation. You may use herbs that are contraindicated during pregnancy:

- Liu Wei Di Huang Wan (Six Ingredient Pill with Rehmannia)—Kidney Yin deficiency.

- Zhi Bai Di Huang Wan (Anemarrhena, Phellodendrom, and Rehmannia Pill)—for early ovulation due to deficient Heat.
- San Er Wu or Si Wu Tang (Four Substance Decoction) + Yin Yang Huo (epimedii) + Xian Mao (curculiginis) + Wu Zi Tang (Five Seed Decoction) (Fu Pen Zi (Chinese raspberry), Gou Qi Zi (Chinese wolfberry), Tu Si Zi (cuscuta), Wu Wei Zi (schisandra berry), Che Qian Zi (plantago seeds))— Blood and Kidney Yang deficiency.
- Dang Gui Shao Yao San (Angelica and Peony Powder)—Liver Blood deficiency, Liver Qi stagnation.
- Tao Hong Si Wu Tang (Four Substance Decoction with Safflower and Peach Pit)—Blood stasis.
- Gui Pi Tang (Restoring the Spleen Decoction)—Spleen Qi and Heart Blood deficiency.
- Tian Wang Bu Xin Dang (Heavenly Emperor's Pill to Tonify the Heart)— Kidney Yin and Heart Blood deficiency.

Luteal phase strategies

Nourish Liver Blood, tonify Kidney Qi, tonify Spleen Qi, harmonize Liver, gently Move and cool Blood; use herbs contraindicated during pregnancy cautiously:

- Bu Zhong Yi Qi Tang (Tonify the Middle and Augment the Qi Decoction)—Spleen Qi deficiency (modified—omit Chai Hu (bupleurum), and add astringents, Tu Si Zi (cuscuta), Ai Ye (mugwort), Chi Shao (red peony), Xu Duan (dipsacus), Huang Qin (skullcap root), etc.).
- Gui Zhi Fu Ling Wan (Cinnamon Twig and Poria Pill)—Blood stasis.
- Dang Gui Shao Yao San (Angelica and Peony Powder)—Liver Blood deficiency.
- Dan Zhi Xiao Yao San (Free and Easy Wanderer)—Liver Qi stagnation with Heat.
- San Er Wu—Ba Zhen Tang (Eight Treasure Decoction) + Yin Yang Huo (epimedii), Xian Mao (curculiginis), Wu Zi Tang (Five Seed Decoction)— for Qi, Blood, and Kidney Yang deficiency.
- Ba Wei Di Huang Wan (Eight Ingredient Decoction with Rehmannia)— Kidney Qi deficiency.
- Wan Dai Tang (End Discharge Decoction) or Yi Huang Tang (Change

Yellow (Discharge) Decoction) modifications—Spleen Qi deficiency (dampness/uterus leakage)—modifying for the actual pattern.

Menstrual formulas to resolve stasis and address painful periods

- Wen Jing Tang (Warm the Menses Decoction).
- Gui Zhi Fu Ling Wan (Cinnamon Twig and Poria Pill).
- Xue Fu Zhu Yu Tang (Drive Out Stasis in the Mansion of Blood Decoction).
- Shi Xiao San (Sudden Smile Powder).

While prenatal formulas will help set the stage for pregnancy, it is important to evaluate the status of the Blood throughout pregnancy, and resume formulas like Si Wu Tang (Four Substance Decoction) and Ba Zhen Tang (Eight Treasure Decoction) as signs of Qi and Blood deficiency manifest.

The internal queendom of the soul

I am the child of the Mother and Father Tao.

Now that we've visited the creative systems life utilizes to manifest itself into this three-dimensional Earth life, let's close this chapter with a story about the journey of the soul and the meaning of life. The Taoists viewed the body symbolically as a sacred internal landscape that the spirits inhabit to experience their earthly curriculum. Every Heart-Mind experiences a different view of life and therefore a different landscape. While we perceive material form with our sensory organs, our inner interpretations are based upon quite another reality altogether. Our perspectives establish the functioning of the entire endocrine system, our inner empire.

The tapestry of the life you've lived is imprinted in the fabric of your body and mind. Your meridians tell the story of your survival: how you've made it this far; what lessons you've learned in your life interactions; and how you define yourself in this moment in time. From the Jing of your given potential, how have you financed your life experiences with your Qi and Blood to give who you think you are meaning?

While Zhuang Zi alluded to the body as a symbolic country in the 4th century BCE, very few written references can be found, and virtually no systematic classification. Yet, as we all know, the *Su Wen* assigns agents to execute the necessary functions to keep the body as a country operating smoothly: the Lungs are the officers of rules and regulations; the Liver is the general that devises strategies; and the Heart, which stores the spirit, holds the office of monarch from whence the spirit light emanates and whose orientation is joy. The body is so much more than a body.

Myths and metaphors provide a picturesque context for the mystic journey of the soul and are meant to evoke a Heart quality that can't be encapsulated by a scientific approach. They are not fixed historical facts; their only valid interpretation is the meaning we each impart by living it out in our own lives. Here, in this soul-growing empire, the inner landscape meets the outer landscape through the interface of the Heart-Mind's interpretations. As we embody our life lessons, the Ling soul is the fabric we create out of the warp of Jing and the weft of the soul's precious thread that comes from the center of the cosmos. Chapter 8 of the *Su Wen* says that these fine threads multiply by the thousands and tens of thousands until they can be weighed and measured, creating the bodily forms. Its colors and textures are provided by the environmental conditions produced by our mental and emotional movements that stir up the Qi. Our virtues are built by the challenges we encounter and overcome on our way home to the Tao.

We begin our journey out of the womb as Jing, which will exchange itself for Qi and Shen. And at our journey's end our Essence will be etched with meaning as we are lifted back into our cosmic nest with a lively story to tell. The illustration of the Nei Jing Tu (Chart of the Inner Warp), originally copied from a silk scroll but presently engraved into a slab on the walls of the White Cloud Taoist Temple in Beijing, tells one such story. Place yourself inside.

The image begins at the base of the sacrum where a young boy and girl play on a waterwheel, gaily exchanging Yin and Yang. Their innocent play, raw and not yet wise, initiates the first chakra pressure that drives our Water energies and Marrow up the spine, the passage of the Milky Way. Its first pass is a fiery cauldron in the low back that creates the Will, and where the churning of Water and Fire produces the necessary alchemy for the soul's many possible transformations.

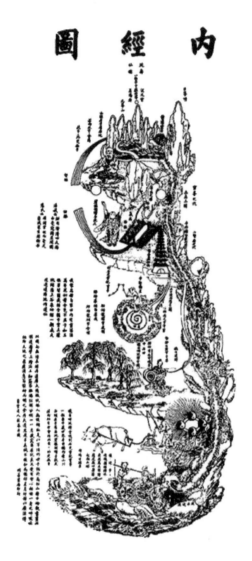

The Nei Jing Tu

A mortal oxherd boy lives in the lower Dan Tien, where he uses his life force assisted by oxen to plow the fields in search of seven coins buried deep within the underbelly. Row after row he digs to uncover these hidden treasures in the rough. Eventually these coins, if rightly valued, will purchase his way through Heaven's gate. His toil is in service to his beloved maiden who occupies the area of the solar plexus, the yellow court where inhabitants come together and where rituals take place.

This weaver girl, also in love with the oxherd boy, is actually immortal, in service to the Queen Mother of the West, Xi Wang Mu (the goddess of life, death, and resurrection prior to 700 BCE), who resides in the mountain peaks of the upper Dan Tien. Xi Wang Mu didn't approve of this union and banished the weaver girl from her heavenly home to the Moon due to her mundane taste for mortal love, but granted her a conciliatory rabbit to keep her company. Now, overseeing fertility on Earth, she governs the lunar cycles and weaves the material of life on her cosmic loom, while waiting for her annual permitted meeting with her love. Union of the intention and Will can produce earthly offspring, or can lead to full integration of the intention and Will in service to Heaven.

The fully integrated self is depicted by a pure, genderless, sage baby, residing in the area below the heart. Those seven coins uncovered by the Will, which purchased the difficult lessons of this earthly existence, have been transformed into gold. The infant sage strings them together to form the Big Dipper, which represents the galactic center and the rebirth of our highest self, both innocent and wise, the embryo of immortality. Yet these coins are not meant to be hoarded; they will purchase entrance into the upper realms where our highest treasure awaits.

A sacred pagoda, 12 stories high (representing manifestation in its fullness), lies at the throat representing the rings of the trachea, through which we breathe and speak. This energetically rich area, nestled between the Windows of Heaven, is the thoroughfare we ascend and descend like a ladder between the heart and the head.

Celestial dew passes beneath Heaven's bridge at the roof of the mouth, where the blue-eyed monk lifts the peach of immortality to Lao Tzu, whose eyebrows sweep away the debris of delusion. The radiance of the sun is the left eye, the obscure brilliance of the moon the right; between them the True Invisible One who must get through the Nine Peaks of the Immortals that tower behind, where Xi Wang Mu (Queen Mother of the West) resides, with eight immortal companions. When the journey is completed, the True authentic one will crystallize and return through the crown of the head to her heavenly home.

Each being takes birth to explore certain curricula in their upcoming life. Each will be provided specific life circumstances and challenges to learn these lessons and thereby reach Heaven's destiny. When we are born into our innocence, these concerns lie hidden and dormant, like seven major issues buried in the gut, and will emerge when life presents situations ripe for their learning. They will be represented by what we love, what we are drawn toward, or what cause us the most challenging issues in life that will weave the specific colors and textures into the fabric of our life story. Their strands can propel us upward, cause knots in the fibers that we can't seem to untie, or drag us down if we don't relate to them rightly. And ultimately the conflicts we don't deal with will be passed on.

The *Su Wen* says that when we speak of antiquity we must link it with the present, here and now in our lives. This Taoist narrative provides an ancient story through which we can recognize our own journey from innocence to wisdom. The Ministerial Fire in the low back seeks redemption, and the Sovereign Fire in the chest seeks dominion; together they propel the soul ever upward from lower to middle to upper Dan Tien. When we reach the celestial dew and the land of immortality, it sets the stage for the entire functioning of the hypothalamus and pituitary gland as well as everything downstream. The clearer we are in our own journey, the smoother our Qi will flow. But make no mistake—this is a two-way journey. We must ever spiral back and return to gather any dormant lessons that remain buried in the hidden recesses that can again take us to ever-higher realms. We don't leave any part of ourselves behind.

Who governs her own body governs the country.

How we live our lives and perceive our world establishes the interaction of the entire body–mind–spirit cosmos. The answers to these questions can definitely impact the functioning of the endocrine system, and the output of reproductive and stress hormones. Ask yourself, or have your clients ask themselves:

- When you look at your own innate innocence, how has it propelled you into a higher understanding?
- Where might you still be childish and lacking wisdom?
- Where is your will directed—in service to fleeting external desires?
- Is anything left over to nourish your inner creative energies?
- What have you woven out of your life up to now, and how have you extracted meaning from it?
- What does the weaver girl represent to you?
- Do you feel any conflict between mortal and divine love?

- Have you ventured into your own underworld to uncover the shadowy realm of the Po?
- What life challenges have turned into treasured lessons?
- What aspects of your life have not been integrated into your heart?
- Do you speak truth more from your heart or your head, and how might it impact thyroid functioning?
- What desires exceed your ability to achieve them?
- What causes your heart to be weighed down?
- Is there any residual sadness you harbor?
- Where do you feel like you are not in sync with your life?
- Are there any parts of yourself that are out of sync?

CHAPTER 3

Preconception Preparation

In the same way we can't do anyone else's healing for them, an acupuncturist can't perform their patient's preconception preparation, either. It is an inside job. The highest level of human attainment is to become authentic. Chapter 39 of the *Su Wen* says that *those who are good at speaking of heaven must have experienced it in humanity…those who are good at speaking of humans must be satisfied with themselves…and through the deep examination of self one can be free of confusion and lift the veil.* As practitioners, we must have a deep understanding of our own lives; then, if we are not blocked within ourselves, we can quietly transmit the power of this deep presence of who we are to another. Only then may it move their spirits and our treatments will be successful. This chapter, therefore, while intended for you, the doctor, will also be applicable for your patients. In the realm of Shen, it's the same.

Before thinking about conceiving anything or anyone, conceive of this: you have been begotten by the cosmic forces that have, since the beginning of humanity, united the Yin and Yang of parental Jing with the heavenly Qi of the cosmos to produce you, this most unique expression of life that ever has been. There is a great price to pay for this most magnificent recognition. You must journey to discover that inmost treasure, the sacred signature written on your soul, and begin to live it. For only then will the prenatal Jing assigned you receive its heavenly influx at the Tian Ji that empower Ming Men to live out your ultimate design.

Edgar Cayce described conception as a channel for the expression of divinity into materiality, and that while ovulation belongs to the laws of nature, "conception is a law of God" (Chopra *et al.*, 2005). Life happens through us, not by us or to us. Since the Qi follows the Heart-Mind, preconception preparation is primarily about the mind's orientation and secondarily about physical preparation. The mindset that seems to be most open to igniting the spark of life is one that has learned to let go and surrender itself to reality and doesn't concern itself with how to control its manifestations. The Metal element, through the Lung and Large Intestine, is responsible for exercising the strength of letting go. This releasing energy governs both menstruation and the Po's manifestation.

Surrender seems opposed to the most popular ideas of how to "intend" something. Most of us have been groomed to believe that if we want something bad enough and we try hard enough to reach our goal, we will attain it through sheer effort. This might be true if your aim is a college degree, a million dollars, or a home on the beach. Just rev up those adrenal hormones, focus your mind on your target, and you are likely to achieve it. Yet, as Zhuang Zi said of the archer who was overly attached to his mark, "The need to win drains him of his power." These competitive and obsessive Yang tendencies may rule our economy and the reproductive medical industry, but they have no business in the energies that govern fertility. We don't "make" babies; nor is fertility a "doing;" it's a deep allowing that happens below everyday consciousness. The goal-oriented hyped-up adrenal stress hormones antagonize fertility. The reproductive system is based upon its receptivity far more than its activity. From the hypothalamus to the pituitary gland to the ovarian hormones and uterine lining, the cells must be receptive. If your objective is to draw a new soul into your life, you are more the target than the arrow. Or, to confuse the metaphor with more of Kahlil Gibran's teaching from "On Children:" *You are the bows from which your children as living arrows are set forth.* And it is the archer's job—with a still and quiet heart—to let go and release.

The character Nei Ren 內 is a person who is inside. This conveys a meaning of being content with the interior spaces. Women are inherently more Yin, more internal. Yet we live in a Yang world where we have lost access to our subtle origins, to the deep meaning of life that is found only within, and our ability to touch into the very process of creation. Instead we *decide* to have children, and *try* to conceive, going contrary to the laws of the miraculous origin. Preconception preparation includes giving responsibility back to the origin. First of all, learn to inhabit your inner spaciousness, where your soul is free to live on purpose.

Desire

Overly focusing on a baby produces conflict in the nervous system. It tells the body-mind, "I am focusing on what's missing," a mindset that shifts the body toward sympathetic nervous system dominance and resultant anxiety. Hurriedness has no place here. More than anything else, the mental urgency about bearing a child prevents it. The character for anxiety 急 shows a hand grabbing a person. It pulls and stirs the heart up and outward, as if fueled by adrenaline. It is also the character for impatience, violence, and irritation—an agitated Yang state that is not conductive to receptivity (and nor is it an ideal environment to grow babies). The distress of wanting and trying impacts not only the Heart, but also the uterus, with which it has difficulty communicating.

We don't *make* babies any more than we willfully made ourselves. We didn't just decide to grow ourselves out of the cosmos, fill in our flesh with bones and organs; and nor did we fill our own minds with the ideas we harbor. While we are self-replicating and have access to the power of creation, we are not self-made, at least in the egoic sense. Nor are we mere happenstance. Planned or unplanned, pregnancies aren't seen as accidental. Held in the mystery of the infinite, we are all here by design not of our own egoic making. The Tao, which does not err, stirs all things into being, and all things, of themselves, naturally go out of being; neither is preferable. Because you are here, you have meaning. It is as simple as that. Not to be figured out, but to anchor you in the mystery beyond comprehension where life flows into being. Worrying about infertility is like worrying about insomnia; we can't make ourselves fall asleep or fall pregnant, but we can develop a mindset where it is more likely to happen. And that is a mindset of receptivity, where the soul resides.

When women start to notice how stressed their systems are by all of their doing, they often ask how to let go. The question actually just cancels itself out. Letting go is not a "how to." Instead, they can start to notice all of the ways they hold on and try to remain in control. Notice all of the thoughts about intending a child, and let them go. Notice all of the little muscular tensions caused by trying and let them go. It seems more couples conceive when they stop trying than those who keep straining to get the equation right. Once their systems are balanced, instead of being ruled by ovulation predictor kits, I recommend they make love when their hearts feel most open. The result is it frees up their energy so the Lungs can descend and aerate the Kidneys.

When we've begun to recognize how attempts to control close us off from the life-giving power of the universe, we can move into the secret of receptivity, a concept quoted in the 12th-century "immortal woman" Zhou Yuan Jing's poem, *The secret of the receptive must be sought in stillness. Within stillness there remains the potential for action...* The secret of the receptive is a Yin state, like a quiet meditative Heart-Mind that can receive the subtle urgings of Heaven because it isn't distracted by the clamor of mental activity working away toward its goal. And this is where the potential for powerful action lives.

But the mind can't focus on concepts like nothing, the infinite mystery, or the unborn eternal birthing place of all that is that never comes into or goes out of being. It fills in the gaps because the Yi still wants something to focus on, and the Zhi to work toward. So as we release and become more receptive, we can attune ourselves to the higher frequency of the vibratory field through which manifestation arises. The *Tao Te Ching* (*Book of the Way*) draws its inspiration from the female principle and urges us to keep to the Yin, yield like Water, and always to return to our true selves. Meditative exercises like this can condition our patients or ourselves to do just that. Relax, exhale, and let's trace the manifestations back to the source.

Meditation

Sit down comfortably, with your tailbone rooted and your crown lifted. Allow your spine to be open, extended, and relaxed. Close your eyes, and as you breathe through your nose, place the tip of your tongue on the upper palate, behind your upper teeth. Focus your breath about two inches below your belly button, the lower Dan Tien. As you inhale, this area should expand and begin to feel warm. At the end of inhalation, root your awareness down to the perineum. As you exhale, let your awareness follow your breath up the spine to the top of your head and back out your nose.

As these steps become one continuous movement, deepen each breath. You may be surprised at how relaxing this process becomes as your energy empties out of your head and into your belly, reducing stress hormones and bringing you to the "water" energies of your body. As your awareness rests in the pelvic basin, the increased Qi and Blood will fill it with a tingling sensation—simultaneously relaxed and vibrantly alive.

In this peaceful state, the cells are more receptive to hormonal messages. The relaxed circular muscles from your eyes, mouth, and throughout the peristaltic movement of the digestive system are allowed to descend fully.

Feel yourself deepen, as if you are sinking to the bottom of the ocean floor.

Here you don't see anything, hear anything, taste anything, smell anything, or touch anything. There is no need for thought. Just rest in the depths of your being. You are. You are here. This naked being is your greatest gift. Keep breathing in and out, slowly, deeply.

Eventually, as the mind quiets down, you may feel that there is no division between inside and outside. In this state of being, you are connected to the source of all. It's hard to tell if you are in the universe or if the universe is within you. The top of your head is connected to "Heaven" or the cosmos. The tip of your tailbone is grounded in the earth. You are in between. This is home, the place to begin and return. It is called the Mysterious Feminine, the Doorway of Heaven and Earth. It is the unitive meeting place of Yin and Yang where you are complete and most you—limitless, timeless, unconditional love and peace. Let the quiet vibrations of the universe use you as it will; if you remain a channel for its arisings it will never run dry.

We can use this process to renew ourselves anytime we are willing to relinquish the old structures and inhabit our core, through which we can recognize the threads of Heaven. The psychic force condenses into energy and with the directional capacity provided by Yi and Zhi, can precipitate into actual form. How can we relate with this energy? We actually don't need to; here, the imagination is unnecessary. We just continue to let the awareness deepen. There is a Heart within the Heart that vibrates with a quiet and crystalline frequency that gives us our unique nature. We inhabit this force with our full attention and let it shine to the furthest reaches of the cosmos in the depths of our being. And in the realm of the unborn, a magical quickening of this pure potential dreams itself into a conscious force, now capable of becoming. We can ride this wave of energy, but we must take care not to try to own or control it—just allow and attend to it with a quiet heart.

Many women are aware of the moment of conception where deep inside they feel an energy surge that has been attracted to their expanded Hearts. And these energies, some subtle, some more obvious, continue at implantation and throughout. Some women who miscarry know the moment the child was no longer present, although there were no physical symptoms. As we let go and deepen our awareness, we can learn to attune to this underground force before and after conception, staying with the subtle energy rather than its manifestations. This is where we know our children, and this is where we are known by the eternal creator.

Many enjoy playing in the realm of the psychic where they can weave stories around who or what wants to manifest. The wave on the verge of becoming a particle, however, lives in all possibilities, and can become anything until it follows the gravitational tendencies of the mind and is fired in the great kiln of manifest existence. When we begin to recognize this process within ourselves, we have access to the threads of Heaven. In the internal realm of the unborn, we can cultivate our higher vibratory energies while releasing those that have become more dense and toxic. The "immortals" were able to intensify and crystallize their highest energy centers in the realm of the eternal here and now. While we love to revere and admire them, we each have the capacity to intensify Shen during this lifetime.

Chapter 65 of the *Hua Hu Ching* says:

The interplay of yin and yang within the womb of the Mysterious Mother creates the expansion and contraction of nature. Although the entire universe is created out of this reproductive dance, it is but a tiny portion of her being. Her heart is the Universal Heart, and her mind the Universal Mind. The reproductive function is also a part of human beings. Because yin and yang are not complete within us as individuals, we pair up to integrate them and bring forth new life. Although most people spend their entire lives following this biological impulse, it is only a tiny portion of our beings as well. If we remain obsessed with seeds and eggs, we are married to the fertile reproductive valley of the Mysterious Mother but not to her immeasurable heart and all-knowing mind. If you wish to unite with her heart and mind, you must integrate yin and yang within and refine their fire upward. Then you have the power to merge with the whole being of the Mysterious Mother. This is what is known as true evolution.

While we may not be in search of enlightenment, every single creative endeavor or health condition will benefit when we can open our Hearts and minds to perceive the quiet whispers from the unborn. Human beings, by using their minds in service to the ego, have become rather dense and self-serving, obscuring the power of Shen. It appears that we are in drastic need of this true evolution. Modern science has discovered that DNA carries ancestral trauma through numerous generations. Likewise, Chinese medicine refers to inherited fetal toxins that impact the Jing. The real work in preparing to conceive includes clearing the ancestral trauma as it manifests in each of our lives. As we are liberated from any sense of victimization, we clean up the constitutional level in our ancestral line. Any traumatic experiences in this life, including birth trauma, are only reflections of the primal wound—being separated from our origin. We are outgrowths of a source field that we may have forgotten but have never lost. Perhaps evolution is calling for humanity to release the density of self, so Heaven can once again open its gates and let life surge.

Sarai was 11 when her mother passed, leaving her to care for her younger brother. At a healing retreat, one week past ovulation, she became aware of how much she resented this role, a profound revelation that freed her from a burden she didn't know she carried. Treating her Chong Mai was in order. As she received her needles in the dimly lit therapy room of the spa, the air became electrified, charged with an energy that made our hair stand on end. Sarai had a sudden seizure like movement, gasped, and laid in a state of peaceful bliss for the rest of her treatment. Afterwards she reported being transported to a dreamlike state, where her mother came to her like an angel carrying a child, which she placed directly in her arms. A warm sensation moved from her heart to her belly. She found herself pregnant a week later.

Tonifying your ancestors: how to influence your lineage by changing your story
Physical: lower Dan Tien

Chinese medicine has a concept called "tonifying the ancestors," whose physical component is represented by the Eight Extraordinary Vessels and the strength of our Essence. This is the push behind our Will or life force. Our Kidney energetics provide the genetic springboard from which its manifestations arise. We can think of Jing like the warp of a loom. The stronger the Jing, the stronger the foundation on which the fabric of life will be woven. When the Jing is weak, one may be unable to weave at all, or the compromised material may give in to structural flaws like frayed weft, potentially resulting in miscarriages, low birth weight, and genetic abnormalities.

To strengthen Jing, we can rest, abstain from overactivity, and reduce stress in our lives, all of which shorten the telomeres and reduce the cells' longevity.

Wu Zi Tang (Five Seed Decoction) for tonifying the ancestors includes Fu Pen Zi (Chinese raspberry), Gou Qi Zi (Chinese wolfberry), Wu Wei Zi (schisandra berry), Tu Si Zi (cuscuta), and Che Qian Zi (plantago seeds), which can be added to other formula to address underlying patterns. Harmonizing stagnant Qi, draining Dampness, clearing Heat, and invigorating static Blood will reduce stressors to the Jing, while tonifying deficient Qi, Blood, Yin, or Yang can build up the Jing reserves. Qi Gong exercises that focus on cultivating the energies in the lower Dan Tien reduce sympathetic overload, return blood flow to the origin, and calm down adrenal hyperactivity, which is antagonistic to our reproductive capacity. When Shen, Qi, and Jing are fully present in the moment, with nothing left out, they strengthen one another.

The Kidneys provide Jing that the San Jiao distributes (unevenly) through the back Shu points, setting up our unique constitution, establishing the life challenges fueled by the Gate of Destiny at Ming Men. One of the ways we can check in on how well we are honoring our own authentic constitutional makeup is to quiet the mind and bring our focus to the lower Dan Tien. In your mind's eye, let a picture emerge of yourself as a small child, as young as you can remember. What is the essential quality of her nature? Just let it leave you with a feeling of something indescribably but unquestionably you.

Interactive: middle Dan Tien

Our ancestral Qi or Zong Qi resides in the chest, closely related to the spirits of the Heart and Lungs. While the Kidney energetics define certain inherited genetic traits that give us our starting point, we also inherit particular leanings that will define how we are likely to respond to a given set of environmental influences. We know trauma is inherited and continues to be expressed many generations later, but we also inherit a whole line of survival strategies that worked. How do we know? We're here. We could call this Zong Qi, the ancestral gathering Qi of the chest, or we could describe the whole process as the study of epigenetics. Together with our constitution, these influences impact how our temperaments will develop.

Returning to the image of your Essence as a small child, bring your awareness now to the center of the chest. The Heart is the locus of a woman's spiritual power, more than her lower Dan Tien. Have these qualities been adequately nurtured, cultivated, or brought to life? How has your behavior been shaped by it—positively or negatively? Working at this level can allow you to maximize positive and overcome negative ancestral influences that have been triggered in your lifetime.

Differentiation: upper Dan Tien

The Kidneys are the body's reproducing machines. Within and without, we reproduce not what we want, but what we are. Taoist images, like that provided by the Nei Jing Tu, depict the right and left Kidneys as a waterwheel and cauldron, played upon by our innate innocence. This movement drives Water up the spinal column and into the Sea of Marrow in the head. Through the eyes, depicted as the inner sun and moon, our brain then reproduces our view of life into how it mutually perceives ourselves, the world, and its inhabitants. The Chinese character Xiang 相 portrays an eye and a tree to represent mutuality. While this pictogram has been described as someone peeking from behind a tree, its deeper meaning of mutual arising is that in the process of seeing, we create the tree. And the tree, in the process of being seen, awakens our eyes. We make the tree, like the world, into what it means for us. As we wake up in the morning, the Hun, who have been resting in the Liver, rise up to the eyes to project our world, as we see it. And this process initiates the entire cascade of endocrine functioning. As we will see later on, the way we uniquely perceive our lives and project the world is established in utero. Figuratively we must return to the womb of the cosmic mother for our vision to be renewed.

The mind is either focused externally or internally. When focused externally, we may get a lot done, but we tend to be thrown around by centrifugal engagements and very little transformation takes place. *The Secret of the Golden Flower* speaks of *turning the light of the dipper around*, which means bringing one's conscious awareness, represented by the Heart, within. This does not mean narcissistic fascination with the content of one's mind, but being present to our own inner landscape, where we may have to encounter some uncomfortable shadows that have been lurking in the dark. If we remain witnesses at this level, we can actually experience the sense of communicating with and "healing" those who have come before us. When one overcomes life issues that have been passed down to us, we end their legacy—we've tonified ourselves, our ancestors, and our children. As you shine the light of awareness within, your own powerful transformative energies can dissolve these negative patterns and resolve them once and for all. The dark can rest. The light then shines on itself, no longer through the prism of our delusions. For each bit of density we overcome, our creations will enter this existence with a higher vibratory level. All imbalances arise from being out of harmony with spirit, and all healing comes from the spirit. This, it seems, is the greatest legacy we can leave in this life.

MOTHERS' PRECONCEPTION GUIDELINES
Nutrition

The best fertility diet is able to provide each individual with the highest energy and the lowest amount of stress to the system. First try to eliminate substances that stress and toxify. Then eat foods that are life- and growth-enhancing.

Reduce or eliminate:

- Caffeine, alcohol, nicotine, and any unnecessary medication
- Artificial colors, flavors, or preservatives
- Sugars, sugar substitutes, and refined carbohydrates
- Packaged, processed, and prepared foods
- Unhealthy trans fats and unnecessary fried foods
- Hormonally treated milk, dairy, and animal products.

Include:

- Organic colorful, soft leafy greens, orange and red vegetables
- Organic fruits
- Seeds, beans, legumes, nuts, and nut butters
- Organic, whole, and non-GMO grains
- Eggs, fish, and organic yogurt
- Organic, non-hormonally treated animal products.

Supplement:

- Iron, folate, vitamin B12, and zinc will help build the blood
- Deep sea fish oil will nourish the Essence, keep the Blood moving, support fetal brain development, and allay postpartum depression.

Lifestyle

- Are you (and your partner) emotionally prepared to raise a new being together?
- Is your living environment conducive to your highest health and wellbeing?
- What people, relational dynamics, work environments, behaviors, and lifestyles are not consistent with the new life you wish to bring forth?
- Is your physical exercise level conducive to carrying another being in your body?
- What are some changes you can make right now?
- What changes are you willing to make next month?
- What changes need to be made but you don't know how to make them?
- Take note of the speed of your life. See if you can find your own internal pace, and adjust your activities to match your internal rhythm.

Physical exercises

- Plant your bare feet on the ground and connect with the energy of the earth. Feel as if you are absorbing the life-giving energy from the center of the earth, drawing it into the bottom of your foot. Draw the energy up into your pelvis as you breathe into your womb.
- A perineal lift can help strengthen and energize the tissues that will support your pregnancy and eventually birthing. Sit in a chair and press the first metatarsal bone (behind your big toe) toward the ground while you simultaneously squeeze and lift the perineum and levator ani muscles. The more you do this, the more tone and control you'll have over your vagina and perineum.
- Practice mobilizing your joints—all of them. Circle your pelvis, hips, ribcage, neck, shoulders, elbows, wrists, knees, ankles, and feet.
- Learn to squat like a woman—our original design made it most efficient to squat when we peed, pooped, and gave birth, and when we did we had far less pelvic dysfunction. With your feet more than shoulder-width apart and your toes pointing out to open your groin, stand like an upside-down Y. Alternate bending one knee at a time

while taking care that the bent knee doesn't extend beyond your toes. When this gets easier, move your feet out further (toes still facing out) and lower your buttocks down as far as is comfortable. Let your inner thighs lift you back up. Repeat until you feel like you've had enough, but not until you are sore. Trust your body.

- Then bring your feet a little closer together, toes ahead, and practice lowering your behind as you feel your thighs holding you up. Try not to let your knees extend beyond your toes. Your back should be as straight as is comfortable, lifting and lowering with the emphasis on your upper thighs, groin, and buttocks. Do not strain or grunt. You have nine more months to master this.

Self-inquiry exercises

The preparatory phase begins when one's longing for life meets the soul's movement toward incarnation. These exercises can begin to bridge the gap between the prenatal and postnatal domains, reducing the sometimes dense wall between that which is unconscious and that which is conscious. The most courageous work you can do is decide to gestate consciously.

As you evaluate each phase of prenatal development, it is natural for uncomfortable feelings to arise where there are unresolved issues. The most opportune time to work through any unhealthy emotional patterns is before they influence future incarnations, not after.

Alignment worksheet

Answering the following questions can stimulate thoughts, feelings, concerns, and parallels you may have drawn—even unconsciously—about pregnancy and childbirth, and where these attitudes originated. Shining the light of awareness within can acknowledge and release conflicting messages:

- What did your mother tell you about her experiences conceiving, carrying, and delivering you?
- What specifically did you hear, or what became your story about your birth?
- Was your mother working at the time of her conception? How old was she? Did she continue what she was doing prior to your birth after you were born?

- Did you represent the fulfillment of her life's dream—or not?
- What did she tell you about it? What feelings does this evoke in you? Have you ever discussed this with her?
- Are you feeling pressure from outside sources (even messages you received from childhood) to bring forth this creation?
- Do you worry about conception, being pregnant, or giving birth?
- What have you heard about pregnancy, childbirth, parenting, or caring for this new creation that creates concerns?

Exploring ambivalence about having a baby

You may feel you are totally ready to conceive on every level, or you may be experiencing fears about becoming pregnant or giving birth (to your creation). We all experience some ambivalence, no matter how excited we are. Some of the issues reside beneath our conscious awareness. The following questions can help clarify any conflicted feelings that may physiologically affect the reproductive process. Becoming aware of all your feelings is the key. Unconscious mixed messages can throw off the delicate balance of the endocrine system. This exercise will help you explore the origin of any ambivalence you may have. Getting in touch with and expressing negative feelings and conflicts frees pent-up emotional energy.

Why I want a baby/child	Why I don't want to have a baby/child
Object of desire	Or the creation I wish to bring forth

- Which reasons are yours alone? Which are your mate's, your mother's, your father's, your siblings', or your friends'?
- Recall the reasons your parents gave for wanting children. Are their reasons similar to yours, or dissimilar? What are your feelings—emotional and physical—when you read your answers to these questions?
- Which positive traits do you think you might pass on to your offspring?

- Which negative traits do you fear you might pass on to them?

According to Chinese wisdom, the gestation period sets up the lessons your child will encounter during their own life path. The five elements contained in these lessons are:

Element	Organ	Emotional extreme	Virtue
Fire	Heart	Elation	Trust
Earth	Spleen	Obsessive thought	Integrity
Metal	Lung	Sadness	Order
Water	Kidney	Fear	Wisdom
Wood	Liver	Anger	Compassion

Minimizing emotional extremes and maximizing virtues can provide your child with a conscious entrance into this life, ideally free of the burdens you have worked through. As much as you can, use this pregnancy to take care of your own life challenges so that you can reduce the baggage you pass on to your child. You can do this by paying attention to the emotional issues that grab hold of you and bringing the light of your own awareness into the shadow of your own subconscious mind. By acknowledging your deepest issues, your pregnancy can become a time to raise your own consciousness vibrations, providing a more positive imprint so your child can enter this world unhindered by your unresolved issues.

Exercise to keep hope alive within

The pure and tender longing to bear new life showers our neurotransmitters with hope. When this arising of the heart is followed loosely, it remains pure. Life longs for more of itself. When grasped too tightly it can easily become a major source of frustration and stress, antagonizing reproductive hormones.

One of the main impediments on the journey toward parenthood is excess desire. At first, desire keeps us hopeful. Ongoing unfulfilled desires can lead to despondency and stagnation. In this exercise, first think about why you want a child. While the most obvious and superficial aspect of this might be to fit into society, to be a mom among moms, to watch your child play, etc., there is something deeper. The origin of all pure longing originates with an invitation to change ourselves, not our circumstances. When you think of yourself with a child, what is it you expect to feel? For some it may be a feeling of unconditional love, or giving life meaning. Spend some time with this. It is less important that you can name it than it is that you can feel it. Let it fill your heart so that you know it and recognize it and can call it up at will.

Part two of this exercise is to remove the image of your future child from what you wish to attain. Free your child of the need to fulfill your desires. Remember, your job is to fulfill their needs, not the other way around. Having already experienced the feeling you are going for, start to live it, enhancing it in all your affairs. This will magnetize things to you that resonate with what's already fulfilled.

How egg and sperm come together

When the expression of love is held as sacred, it changes the atmosphere that invokes conception. If the Heart isn't in it, sex on command produces a lower vibration. While it may still feel good and get the job done, it may not invoke the most optimum frequency to call in new life potential. If timed sex according to ovulation predictor kits has been your pattern, practice connecting with your partner, and letting your Heart determine when it is time to open. In most cases, women are naturally more receptive around ovulation. All of life is naturally drawn to higher levels of love, joy, and ecstasy.

Querying the soul

Bring your awareness to your heart and feel it start to open, as if it opens up to occupy your entire body. Then see it extend beyond your body and fill up the room you are in. Allow it to move beyond the walls and past the building, the neighborhood, the town, the state, the country, the world, the solar system, and the cosmos.

When you feel expansive enough, query the soul of your future incarnation.

Open your consciousness to the universal wisdom that knows all. If it feels silly at first, keep practicing it; with patience, answers will come. If you'd like to use some prompters:

- Are there any unresolved emotional issues that I need to resolve before I can be fully receptive?

- Is there any friction or discord in my life that I need to resolve before I can be fully receptive?
- Are there any lessons that I need to overcome before I am ready to receive?
- Are there any lessons that my partner needs to resolve before we are ready to receive?
- Is our professional or living situation conducive to this incarnation?
- Do I experience any limits to accepting myself as capable of caring for a child?
- Do I have expectations of a child that are unreasonable?
- Is any aspect of my image of a child inconsistent with an unconditional acceptance of life?
- What life lessons do I need to resolve so I don't pass them on?
- Will I be able to accept and love fully if we are presented with physical, mental, or emotional limitations that may not fit my image of how I'd like a child to look?

What are you reproducing?

Oh, the things we reproduce—ten thousand times a day we birth and rebirth cells, thoughts, habitual movements, and belief patterns. Pay attention to where your reproductive energies are going. Are you rehashing past regrets and playing out future anxieties? What percentage of your daily movements are habitual repetitions of the past? Look at your daily life and see how much new life you have infused into each day. Take note of how often you inhabit yourself and this moment fully. When lost in thought, return to your breathing. Get your Qi and Blood out of your head and back in your body. This is how you can give yourself to the unborn.

PART II

OCCUPYING THE PALACE

The Trimester Model

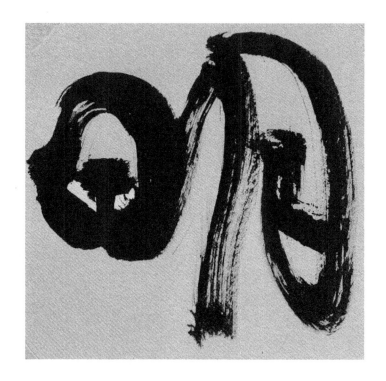

When the time comes for the embryo to receive the spirit of life,
at that time the sun begins to help.
This embryo is brought into movement,
for the sun quickens it with spirit.
From the other stars this embryo

received only an impression,
until the sun shone upon it.
How did it become connected
with the shining sun in the womb?
By ways hidden from our senses:
the way whereby gold is nourished,
the way a common stone becomes a garnet
and the ruby red,
the way fruit is ripened,
and the way courage comes
to one distraught with fear.

—*Rumi, "The embryo,"* 胚胎

The character above is Pei Tai. Pei means embryo and Tai is its expression as a fetus. Together they signify origin. Pei is a coagulated germ of procreation whose pictogram includes a vertical line depicting the human bridge between Heaven and Earth; a slash representing the vectors of wind that signify our impermanent, ever-changing nature; and a drop of dew exemplifying the tears we shed as we accept this ever-changing life of challenges, regrets, our inevitable demise, and another chance at life and renewal. The embryo is our resurrection.

The oldest book of embryology is *The Guan Zi*, or the *Book of Master Guan*, from the 4th century BC:

The person is composed of Water. The Jing of the man and woman unite. Subsequently the Water streams and then makes the form...

At three months it has undifferentiated form...

The five yin organs are now formed, then the flesh is created. The spleen creates the diaphragm. The lung creates the bones. The kidney creates the brain. The liver creates the skin. The heart creates the flesh.

We will draw from the *Taichanshu, Book of Gestation and Birth*, from the Mawangdui manuscript, which, according to Sabine Wilms, predates 168 BCE, and provides advice for caring for the pregnancy month by month.

The physician Chao Yuanfang, from 610 AD, published the *Zhu Bing Yuan Hou Lun (Treatise on the Causes and Manifestations of Diseases)*, in which the progression of the developing fetus is described, which is identical to Sun Si Miao's *Qian Jin Yao Fang* (*Thousand Golden Essential Prescriptions*) from 652 AD. They describe how to manage the pregnancy, and what to expect as the fetus proceeds from the first through to the last of the ten months.

The *Huai Nan Zi* (*The Masters/Philosophers of Huainan*), written in 122 BC, gives a similarly complete embryologic theory from which we will also borrow. The seventh chapter is devoted to describing how life comes into being through Jing Shen. It begins with the beginning:

> Of old, in the time before there was Heaven and Earth:
> there were only images and no forms.
> All was obscure and dark, vague and unclear, shapeless and formless,
> and no one knows its gateway.

Chapter 7.1 goes on to say that *two spirits established Heaven and Earth…differentiated into Yin and Yang; the turbid vital energy became creatures; the refined vital energy became humans*. And, like most Taoist writings, it goes on to speak about the meaning of life before it describes its process of coming into being. Sages take:

> Heaven as father, earth as mother, Yin and Yang as warp, the four seasons as weft. Through the tranquility of Heaven, they become pure. Through the stability of Earth, they become calm… Tranquility and stillness are the dwellings of spirit like illumination; emptiness and nothingness are where the Way resides. For this reason, those who seek for it externally lose it internally; those who preserve it internally attain it externally as well.

Now that the groundwork is laid, Chapter 7.2 launches into a discourse on embryology, beginning with a quote from the *Tao Te Ching* (*Book of the Way*):

> The one generates the two, the two generate the three; the three generate the myriad things. The myriad things carry the yin and embrace the yang and through the blending of vital energy, become harmonious.
>
> Therefore it is said:

> In the first month, fertilization occurs.
> In the second month, a corporeal mass develops.

In the third month, an embryo forms.

In the fourth month, the flesh is produced.

In the fifth month, the muscles form.

In the sixth month, the bones develop.

In the seventh month the fetus forms.

In the eighth month, the fetus starts to move.

In the ninth month, its movements become more pronounced.

In the tenth month, the birth occurs.

The chapter elaborates on five spheres of vital energy, and how they parallel the forces in nature. *The pulmonary orb parallels the air; the hepatic orb parallels the wind...*and then goes on to describe further how we are to live life to conserve and maximize our Quintessential Spirit (Jing Shen).

The Classic of Birth, the grand basis of the *Yellow Emperor's Inner Canon*, says:

The Yellow Emperor asked: "How are humans born?" To that, Qi Bo replied, "To be born, humans are first conceived in the mysterious depth; that is where they first take form in the internal cavity. If such form takes place without disruption, then the human being is conceived. In the first month of pregnancy, it is called a 'pre-embryonic substance', or 'a spore.' The second month it is called embryo. In the third month it develops blood vessels, in the fourth month procures bones, in the fifth month it moves, in the sixth month it takes shape, in the seventh month it grows hair, in the eight month it acquires vision, in the ninth month the grains enter its stomach. In the tenth month the infant is delivered."

Chinese medical thought gave painstaking attention to this topic. We, in our reductionist modern Western view of life, where complexity reigns supreme, continue to debate about when life actually begins and when an embryo constitutes a real human being. We get excited as we see the embryo taking on parts throughout gestation: *now its fingers and toes are formed...*whereas in the Chinese view the embryo is whole from the onset. While it complexifies throughout uterine life, it starts out full and complete, directly from the One. A Taoist view might even say that there is no true "beginning" of life, just a continuation of eternal becoming. The embryo symbolizes the pinnacle of self-cultivation where we can return to a state of our original perfection and union with the source, a state known as the unborn. Gestation is a cosmic event, where the embryo is fashioned in the likeness of the macrocosm. Its head is round like Heaven, and its feet are shaped just for the Earth. We, in the likeness of Heaven and Earth, can return to this cosmic body to cultivate longevity and spiritual culmination at any time. Or, better yet, we never have to leave its domain.

Trimester model

> The Tao gives birth to the One.
> The One gives birth to the Two.
> The Two give birth to the Three.
> The Three give birth to limitless potential.

The trimester theory is the oldest model of pregnancy, originating with the *Tao Te Ching*'s (*Book of the Way*) description of the trinity that underlies life. Tao is the Origin and One is Spirit—consciousness wishing to experience life. Two is the male and female principles whose Jing provides both their DNA and the cumulation of experiences necessary for the advancement the soul. When these come together, the limitless potential will be wrapped so it can sprout into form. Just like Jing and Shen, the embryo and its wrapper are not separate. While the three give birth to all things, all things can be reduced to three; and the three are, of, course, actually one. The three trimesters symbolically represent the elements associated with the Blood: Earth, Fire, and Wood. Here, in this soul-growing place, three aspects of the soul are programmed prenatally:

- First trimester—Po (Earth): *The Tao gives birth to the One.* During the first trimester, Earth banks the form that will provide the Ling soul its basic physical structure. The initiating energetics belong to the lower Dan Tien. From the deathless celestial realm, the journey begins as spirit enters form; the Po spirit is ignited by the friction created through the parents' Jing, the macrocosm becomes the microcosm, and is banked into manifestation around Heaven's blueprint (Original Penetrating Vessel). The first trimester establishes the primal structure upon which the unique character of the soul will be imprinted in the second and third trimesters.
- Second trimester—Shen (Fire): *The One gives birth to the Two.* Governed by the middle Dan Tien, the Shen receives its curriculum—the Po soul

has accepted life through the form of an embryo, and the initial structures are complete. The original nature, as star seedling, has been wrapped in a physical body like free birds now enclosed in a casing. As the soul graduates into the fetal form, Heaven shapes the curriculum of how the child will interact with others and the world, and the unique challenges it will encounter in its upcoming life so it can redeem Shen from its Essence. The unique strengths and weakness are woven into the Source Qi to be distributed and stored in the Blood, providing the beautifully textured fabric of this individual life.

- Third trimester—Hun (Wood): *The Two give birth to the Three.* The final act of our creation story is governed by the upper Dan Tien that establishes how the curriculum will be carried out through time. The Hun expresses time as the smooth flow of Qi. Here, the environment in utero deeply programs the fetus' emerging consciousness. It is exposed to and affected by the weather of its amniotic internal world. Like the unique markings in the rings of a tree, our fetus receives the completion of creation's finishing touches before it emerges into the world to differentiate itself.

CHAPTER 4

First Trimester—Po (Earth)

THE TAO GIVES BIRTH TO THE ONE

Undifferentiated, wriggling...
on the verge of desiring to be born and flourish
but not yet forming.

—Huai Nan Zi, Chapter 2.1

The first trimester, governed by Earth, establishes the blueprint on which the mandate of Heaven, Tian Ming, will be carried out. Chong Mai is that blueprint, which unites the Conception and Governing Vessels. Chong Mai wraps together the spiraling genetic sequence of the Jing and will bank the Qi and Blood to support the Jing's ascent from Ki 11 Henggu (Pubic Bone) to the shoreline of the mysterious gate at Ki 21 Youmen (Hidden Gate). This ascending process represents movement from the dark into the light, and its starting place begins where Jing is etched into the physical blueprint the Po soul will be occupying, referred to as Jing Po.

Po is the corporeal soul responsible for manifesting our very physical being. The earliest word for soul was revealed in bronzeware script dating from as early as 1500 BCE, which referred to Po as lunar brightness. Similar to the pictogram for Ling 靈, Po conveyed the canopy of the sky sending down four raindrops from Heaven along with a crescent moon and a crowned shaman receiving the celestial light. Unlike the Yang sun, the light from the moon illuminates things in the dark. It gives us access to a deeper wisdom, accessible when the dominance of logical linear thinking dips below the horizon and a different type of embodied wisdom emerges with access to sub- and super-conscious realms. The character for Ming 明, the brightness of illumination, is composed of Rì 日 the character for sun and Yuè 月 the character for moon. Lunar brightness shows up in the right eye, and in GB 24 Riyue (Sun and Moon). The inner light, along with the ability to see in the dark, has been an innate gift of Yin long neglected by our Yang-dominant modern world. We have come to favor, in fact, worship, the external light and the gods of Yang while our internal light has paled. The time has come to turn the light around, and become familiar with the true life-giving capacities of the Mysterious Mother and her cohorts. While it is a woman's birthright, frankly, now it has become a command.

Po is the soul of embodiment that governs the first trimester of pregnancy. During the first three months of gestation, the ancestral spirit of the mother provides the organizing principle to create the entire physical structure. Here in our inner basin, the first five units of Chong Mai from Ki 11–16 are emblematic of our undigested, unprocessed, shadowy issues, like shame (belongs to the Stomach) and guilt (belongs to the Lungs). These antagonize the Kidney's sense of trust in our own ability and eat away at the Jing. Until these issues are resolved, they will be repeated or reproduced, into children, or cancerous growths.

Po is how our inmost being is fearfully and wonderfully *knit together in our mother's womb* (borrowed from Psalm 139). Similar to the first primal meridian, the Conception Vessel, Po provides the animating spirit of autonomic functions that give rise to breathing, suckling, digestion, peristalsis, excretion, balance, proprioception, and the opening and closing of the pores. Lorie Dechar's *Five Spirits* (2006) provides the best description of Po I've come across:

The po is the yin, materialized aspect of the soul. In the macrocosm of the mountain, the po spirits are discovered beyond the dark gate that leads to the caves and labyrinths in the underworld. Deep in the darkness of the caves, amidst the minerals, stones and decaying compost of matter, the po spirits exist in a state of half-slumbering silence. The po are the animating agents of vital life processes that take place beyond our conscious awareness and control. They are closely related to the autonomic nervous system, the sensory receptors—especially the primitive touch responses of the skin—and the interior sense receptors of the visceral organs...the po and the zhi can be correlated with more primitive aspects of the brain such as the limbic system and cerebellum.

According to Lorie Dechar's extensive research and work with the Po souls, it wasn't until the more modern Hun concept entered between 475 and 220 BCE that the Po began to be viewed as problematic. Before that time, when the Mysterious Mother was the origin, the Po were seen to deliver messages from the dark goddess. The Po soul belongs to Xi Wang Mu (Queen Mother of the West), the goddess of life, death, and renewal, who governed descent and resurrection not only of the moon, but also of our own constantly rejuvenating souls. Prior to 700 BCE Xi Wang Mu was known as the Tiger Mother and she guided those courageous enough to surrender to the underworld into true transformation.

As we are brought into renewal and rebirth, we are often asked to relinquish something old and worn out. It might be something we treasure, like an eye, representing our previous way of viewing ourselves and life. Think of Odin's sacrifice at Mimir's Well at the roots of Yggdrasil, the world tree in Norse mythology. As we walk with the Mysterious Mother into the alchemist's crucible, the turbid creature energy becomes refined into something most precious, like a jewel at Jing Ming, and we see a little brighter.

Po, the soul's lunar whiteness responsible for growth, is the same Po as the waxing and waning moon, whose subtle cues urge us inward. One of the variants of Po was associated with the dark aspect of the moon, where our inner light enters into the void that feels like a black hole containing our psychic dregs. These are the neglected or rejected parts of the initial wounding we take on when we consent to separating from the Tao in order to be born. They might cause our animal body to feel drawn inward and depressed, to become enraged or impassioned, or to make us feel as if we are possessed. They might be leftover hauntings from the past or tangled emotional issues that somehow got caught in the body. The Po can be recognized by their downward pull, as if to draw Shen into the neglected underworld.

The Po represent our attachments to things that keep us bound to Earth. And we are greatly attached to our bodies. One of our most terrifying fears is that we *are* the body, since we know it is going to give out one day. If our Po lessons are overcome, we no longer identify only as the body, which casts the shadow of all of our suffering. This includes our unrealized dreams and unresolved issues over which we feel stuck, ashamed, or guilty, where the Po remain lodged inside the body. Unable to leave, they become the Gui (ghosts) that haunt us. Our only remedy is to meet them with compassion so they can be understood and forgiven. When we come to recognize these internal hauntings, we can feel their lodging place in the body-mind, name them, see their value, and thank them for their lessons so their dregs may be released through Po Men. But their gifts remain, like gems under pressure, waiting for us to dig them up and shine them. Unfinished business and unresolved grief prevents the Lungs from descending to the Large Intestine so these issues can be relinquished. Lu 2 Yunmen can dispel murky issues so the Lung Qi can descend. But do not try to banish them. If we try to get rid of them without learning their lessons, they will re-emerge, sometimes with a vengeance. Because the Qi flows with the mind, it follows that if we relate to the Po as demonic, it will only produce further states of dis-ease. Without the Po, the Jing would be inert. We need them. While the Shen allow all perception, the Po grant us physical sensation. Not only do they provide the instincts to keep us alive; they allow us to feel. Mary Oliver's poem "Wild Geese" begins with what I consider to be an apt description of healthy Po:

> You do not have to be good.
> You do not have to walk on your knees
> for a hundred miles through the desert, repenting.
> You only have to let the soft animal of your body
> love what it loves.
> Tell me about despair, yours, and I will tell you about mine...

A funeral banner of Lady Dai Xin Zhui from the 2nd century BCE was discovered at Mawangdui. It is woven with rich imagery of the seven Po souls coming in and going out, revealing the soul's journey through the earthly realm. Lady Dai's banner depicts the summons of the soul and its voyage back to Heaven. At the bottom lies the netherworld of eternal darkness, where water creatures emerge from the cosmic womb, and where the soul undergoes its first metamorphosis. The upper portion illustrates the journey of her soul, accompanied by creatures both worldly and otherworldly—tortoises, birds, and dragons—as she is drawn toward a sun and moon that represent the supernatural light of her own immortality. Two deities of destiny hold the record of her life and guard the entrance through which she must pass into the celestial realms. Emblematic of the rich imagery of the Tian Ji—the threads from Heaven prior to materialization that hook onto the Ming—the soul's golden thread from the center of the cosmos comes with us as we venture forth. While we may not have developed the subtle perception to recognize it, it is there to lead us, especially when we feel we have lost our way. We each similarly weave our own funeral banner through every step of our worldly life. Those who live consciously close to death also live closest to life.

Another view of Po's life lessons, perhaps a little more graphic, comes from *Zhubing Yuanhou Lun* (*Origin of the Etiology of Disease*). Written around 600 CE by Chao Yuanfang to empower the reader to prevent states of disease, very little acupuncture or herbal medicine was prescribed, but Tao Yin exercises, dietary recommendations, and the importance of following guidance received from nature. The 18th scroll said that every human being is born with thousands (in fact 80,000) of "corpse worms"—inadequacies and imbalances that dispirit or violate us. These resident demons or deities (depending on how you relate to them) are the descendants of the original ancestor that lie dormant in the bowels until the correct environment awakens them.

Not only do these invisible organisms thrive in sweet and fermented environments, the three siblings feed off and represent our three major addictive issues that plague humanity—physical lusts (Lower Jiao), stubbornness and gluttony (Middle Jiao), and greed or ambition (Upper Jiao)—which control the host-like parasites. These germs can be teachers, however—not evils—but will gnaw away and consume the Jing until the curriculum is met. Meanwhile, the Hun report one's karmic progress to the Heavenly Emperor every 60 days like a cosmic report card, sometimes returning with symbolic or troubling dreams from the collective to provide cosmic guideposts to show us how we're caught in the wheel of transmigration in the world of personal, everyday triviality, out of which the microorganisms can propel us toward our soul's immortality. Those we can see are referred to as Chong; those we can't see Gu; those that produce bizarre behavioral changes Gui; and the ones that are flat out demonic, Mo. These don't imply that some are good and some are bad; they describe a spectrum of recognition, which is part of our curriculum, and describe how the Shen respond. These critters lurking latently within our depths can cause symptoms, but like all symptoms, they are reminders of something we are meant to overcome on our evolutionary journey. When we tune within and see where there is some residual confusion or we're out of alignment we can change the internal landscape, and allow them to leave. If we only target the symptoms or try to kill off the organisms, we haven't learned the lesson that will shift consciousness and its inner environment. They'll be back again another time, with a heightened learning experience. But when they're done with us, we no longer identify with them, nor they us. They've devoured what they came for and may exit.

While there are nine types of worms that correspond to our hunger to satiate the nine Heart pains along the soul's journey (which we'll focus on in the second trimester), seven is the number associated with Qi and Gui (ghosts). Since we are in the realm of the Po, let's return to the seven metal coins buried in the gut. These represent hidden or latent issues associated with the seven Po deities: Yin and Yang, Jing, Qi, Shen, longevity and sex, all instincts for survival, security, and socialization. Meant to drive us to survive and thrive, they can also go awry and drive us to addiction, ruin, or madness. One of the ways our Po become hauntings is to resist them, keeping them buried in the turbidity of the Lower Jiao. *The turbid vital energy became creatures; the refined vital energy became humans*, says the *Huai Nan Zi*. Because the Po carry our animal nature, and because we often resist our own animal-like origins, the Po often represent the hidden, rejected, or neglected parts of ourselves. Unexamined, they go underground where they remain latent, only to decay and produce problems later on when our Jing, Qi, and Blood weaken our ability to hold their unresolved nature at bay. As they emerge, they can manifest with inflammation, reactivity, and autoimmune presentations. The reason this is so important for our discussion is because the energetics of conception and implantation center on how smoothly the mother's Po soul receives the incoming Po soul. And gestation takes a toll on Jing, Qi, and Blood. When her unresolved issues come into friction with the embryologic Po, they can create symptoms that dominate the first trimester. Po issues can manifest with symptoms of intense skin sensations like goose flesh and itching, odd rashes, and vague feelings of unrest that accompany and exacerbate other unexplainable physical expressions.

If you haven't had the opportunity before now, use this primal time of renewal to turn the rough base metals hidden in your own underbelly into the golden coins that make up the stars of the Big Dipper constellation in the middle Dan Tien when your lessons are learned. These lessons aren't like the type you learn in school, and letter grades aren't given. The raw material is found within. Your deepest urges are meant to propel you toward your true destiny. Only then can the alchemist's furnace refine the base metal into gold. When the seven gold coins are strung on the golden heavenly thread from the center of the cosmos, you may purchase entrance into the nine peaks in the upper Dan Tien. Just be willing to enter into the school of your own soul, where the radical healing of compassion and forgiveness are its promise. Our goal isn't to take on more knowledge but to empty ourselves of unresolved baggage so it will no longer be recreated—through our body, mind, and life. Only the unencumbered soul can traverse the Nine Peaks of the Immortals. And that which you overcome in your own journey will establish the starting point and potential reach of your offspring. Reach, my friend. Reach. You have everything you need within.

Let your bending in the archer's hand be for gladness;
for even as He loves the arrow that flies, so He loves also the bow that is stable.

—*Kahlil Gibran, "On Children"*

While there are other more complex descriptions of the Po and all of their demonic potential, those that seem to resonate with modern consciousness go along with the seven emotional extremes, seven temptations, and seven deadly sins. It isn't so important that we come up with a particular system to define them, because they are all unique in each one of us. We give them their meaning. Their commonality is that they give rise to vague feelings or troubling issues that produce negativity in the body, representing our subconscious hauntings— basically, issues that haven't yet been consciously recognized. They may come from past trauma giving rise to depression, suffering, and acting out through various addictions. If we can relate to them, however, as lessons—imprinted in utero and triggered by epigenetic circumstances that shape the trajectory of our lives—we can see them as the curriculum we are here to learn. Now we can enter into their domain with a different attitude.

We can relate to the Po as wild and spirited animals lost or trapped in the inner landscape. Animals lack the ability to mentally step outside themselves. Purely physical, they experience the immediacy of this moment without dragging around a past or future self. Humans, however, are endowed with the ability to mentally step outside themselves, see themselves as from without, and separate from their physicality. While this may allow us to see ourselves in third person, it also gives us an experience of being separate and segmented, to see ourselves as entities created by mental images of the past projected into a future where we'll eventually die. The mind's ability to perceive itself as separate from the whole gives rise to our deepest sorrow, and our meanest acting out. Wild animals don't necessarily respond to "Here, kitty kitty," and nor do they care all that much what we think about them. However, when we quiet ourselves and enter their domain, they may reveal themselves. To come back into relationship with the Po, we need to get out of our heads and back into our bodies. Qi Gong exercises are one of the best ways not only to nourish the Jing but also to relate with our Po. Sit down or stand up and breathe. Pay attention to what your body is experiencing and attend to the subtle energies you experience flowing through your system.

Now that we have covered Po issues that tend to dominate the first trimester, we can explore how the physical structures necessary for survival will be laid down. As Po is being banked by Earth during the first three months of gestation, the embryo's development will proceed, utilizing mother's Liver, Gallbladder, and Pericardium energies. During the particular month that each is active, the rule of thumb is that we don't needle that channel unless we must. For example, if during the first month the mother is experiencing tremendous Liver Qi stagnation, we may try to employ GB 34 Yanglingquan (Yang Mound Spring) or GB 40 Qiuxu. If the Qi doesn't spread and her pulse remains wiry, only then consider Moxa or gently needling Lv 3 Taichong (Great Surge).

MOTHERS' GUIDELINES FOR THE FIRST TRIMESTER
Physical Po meditation

The Po speak to us through moods and body sensations—not so much through thoughts and emotions. Decide to attend to the Po spirit at least once a day. Find a quiet time to be with the sensations in your body. Sit down in a safe and quiet place, and start to take in the terrain of your animal body with an attitude of curiosity. You might begin by bringing your awareness to the center of your head, past all of your thoughts. Let an inner light drop down your neck through the chimney of Heaven and into the body. Practice noticing sensations in different areas. You can scan top to bottom, outside to inside, left and right, just noticing. As *The Secret of the Golden Flower* encourages, reverse the handle of the Big Dipper and drop your awareness inside the body. The inner eye is equipped with spiritual night vision that can see in the dark. Where is your attention drawn? Allow it to linger and trust the body's guidance.

Whenever a nagging or gripping feeling arises, first pause. Breathe deeply until you can relax into it. Resist the habit to tell a story about what it means, or to try to make it go away. Psychology will get you nowhere. Try to keep your attention below the neck as you go within and query the feeling. Let its qualities emerge. How does it compare with the rest of your body sensation?

What are its textures and colors? Is there a temperature associated with it? Is it lighter or more dense? As you become familiar with it, enter into the sensation. Query if it represents something (be careful not to insert your own mental story here). Does it feel like it is there for a reason? Does it want to be there? Does it want to leave? Does it know how to leave? Does it need or want anything? If so, can it find a part of your body that can provide it? Continue to stay with the sensations until the process resolves on its own. Perhaps close with a blessing of thanks to Xi Wang Mu (Queen Mother of the West).

Mental Po exercise

Oh, the things we reproduce! A thought passes through consciousness—a sweet longing for a new possibility—and we give it attention. We have just birthed a new arising, and it unwraps itself like the acorn in the dark, fertilized by underlying energies (like fear we won't get what we most want) that live mostly below the level of consciousness. We don't get rid of our anxieties by focusing on the positive; we give birth to them. For every positive thought we attempt to grasp hold of, its equal and opposite resides deeper within.

Elaborating on our desire exercise...the most superficial level of desire sees only what we want: *I want a healthy child, free of any malady or malformation.* Of course we want this outcome, what parent wouldn't? If we wish to unpack it a little bit, however, we can find something deeper. What is it that we hope to feel when we attain the object of our desire, and what would we experience if it didn't turn out as we hoped? Let's say we want to experience unconditional love, and maybe we don't think we can unconditionally love anything other than our idea of perfection. This unchallenged assumption can perpetuate ideas of conditional love and mask our capacity for something much greater. Let's try an exercise to challenge this idea. Can you call up that feeling of unconditional love right now? If the answer is yes, great—keep circulating that feeling so that your child can bathe in its protection.

But what if the answer is no? What if your ability to unconditionally love something less than perfect is missing? Let's not stop here. There's something lurking underneath upon which a higher light can shine so that our unborn child doesn't carry this burden.

The seeds of authenticity are often planted in the dark.

Perhaps the deeper we go we just find more of the absence of unconditional love. Now we are in new, uncharted territory. Perhaps we perceive that our desire for a child is more like a phantom or a ghost of something that we want because we experience it as missing. Instead of love we find the feelings we most want to get away from—perhaps we feel horribly imperfect or immensely lonely and incapable of real love, and we engender more of the same. Remember, we reproduce what we are, not what we want. And we are a conglomerate of our entire ancestry that has come before us, with all of its goodness and badness. We take life in this dimension to experience the duality of positive and negative. We often turn our back on the negative, highlighting our perfections and hiding our imperfections, and when we turn around and dare to look, we usually find fear of our own inadequacy. What if we aren't up to the task of love that's required?

It takes a lot of Wei Qi to keep our fears in hiding. And fear, as we know, not only depletes the Jing; it corrodes it. Fear makes the Qi descend, while worry obstructs the Spleen's ascent, and can complicate, if not cause, many physical issues that arise during the first trimester. If the light is turned around, however, we can begin to recognize these fearful thoughts and ideas and diminish their contracting power. Only then do we have the energy to maximize the good. When we become aware of our own latent issues that corrode the Jing, we resist trying to change, fix, or discard. We recognize them and welcome them like a mother would. Only then are they free to exit.

Po self-inquiry

- Yin Po guards the Kidneys and governs the lower Dan Tien. This is the Po of fright; it provides rest and allows us to go into the darkness. When distorted, it gives rise to selfish desires for pleasure. Where do you find greed, envy, and covetousness in your own life?
- Yang Po guards the Heart and connects us with trust and faith. While anxiety is its emotion, when distorted, it gives rise to unbridled passions. What issues in your life cause you guilt or shame? Where have you sought happiness through material gain?
- Shen Po guards the Lung, the breathing process, grief, and tears. When distorted, it holds on by repressing. Are there issues of your past that haven't been released? Anything where you still feel victimized?
- Qi Po guards the Spleen, thought, and the ability to empathize. When

distorted, we might act out of our authentic nature. Where have you lacked integrity and acted out arrogantly or with pride?

- Jing Po guards the Liver, imagination, the ability to dream, and anger. When distorted, one becomes lost in fantasy or tries to blanket rageful extremes. Are there any issues that overly occupy your daydreams? Where have you or do you express hostility or anger?

- Longevity Po guards the Kidneys and carries fear, and synchronizes us with the natural cycles of life and death. When distorted, our energy might be caught in the past or future, robbing us of this moment. Where have issues of your past not worked out for you? What do you regret? How do you try to protect your youth?

- Sex Po guards the Heart and its happiness, and connects it to the drives of the lower Dan Tien. When distorted, it can sever the Heart–Kidney axis, and divorce sex from a healthy and intimate relationship with self or other. Where have you acted out to satisfy your instinctual drives? Where has your sense of self been disconnected from your heart?

Once you see these issues, they move from inside and are now in front of you instead. Feel free to journal about them, talk to a trusted friend about them, and shake or move any stagnation associated with them out of your body.

CHAPTER 5

Liver: Lunar Month One

Weeks 1–4

Cycle day 1–28

> Jing and shen are received from heaven, subsequently the form and body are received from earth. Therefore it is said one creates two, two creates three, three creates the myriad things. The myriad things carry yin on their backs and embrace yang in their arms. Using harmonious qi it creates harmony. Therefore it is said: In the first month there is gao...
>
> —*Huai Nan Zi, Chapter 7*

The first phase of any new endeavor sets the preparatory stage for how the pre-heavenly realm will be made manifest. As we enter the first phase of the soul's incarnation, new life is dreamed into existence as Wood energies supply the life Blood through which the glimmer of the thing hoped for gains substance. The Liver halts menstruation and redirects the Blood to nourish the developing embryo as it makes its first impression in the world of form.

The first month of pregnancy actually begins on day one of the menstrual cycle, when the palace begins its preparation by shedding the contents of the previous cycle. While we might be conditioned to think that pregnancy begins when we have a positive pregnancy test, it does not. The formation of the embryo begins with an "inkling from above," and is intimately intertwined with the formation of its new home. We actually can't trace the origin of its arising; it goes back to the very first mother. Creator, creation, and the creative process are all one thing. The Chinese view is that one's life begins a year prior to actual birthing, which goes along with our modern understanding of how the germ cells are chosen, prior even to conception.

Let's return to our ritual container, the relational dynamic of a couple in the highly charged field of love. They are like priests and priestesses that surrender themselves to the cosmic principle as their sexual fluids combine. The friction of opposites creates a specific vibration, like a lightning bolt that invokes the third energy, which precipitates into form from the heavenly realms.

Primed for three months, bathed in the fluids of the mother, the follicle finally reaches its apogee. Like volcanic plume, the ovule spills forth from her ovarian home, plunging into the void of the pelvic basin where the fimbrae of the fallopian tube, like Shang Di's hands, sweep her toward the palace of creation. But first, like all new beginnings, she must descend into the mysterious pass, letting go of all moorings to her previous abode. Yet she is not lost. All beings have an inner north star or polestar (Ba Ji) around which the axis of our lives plays out; and the ova, too, have been found to be polarized, from which an energetic field emanates. Knowing nothing of her future, yet daring to come forth anyway, she proceeds into the great unknown down the passageway of the oviduct.

Fertilization

Meanwhile, a force like the Milky Way spirals forth in the corridor of the palace of the child, where millions of knights have ejected on a suicide mission to merge with their queen and be taken into the cosmic womb. The relative scale from ejaculation to fertilization has been likened to the distance from the earth to the moon. Only a few hundred will make it to the goal, goaded on by chemoattractant chemicals that have been excreted by the corpus luteum. The ovum will attract the genetic material most complementarily opposite her own, which will increase the odds of survival. She will select from X female-producing sperm that are more durable and long-lasting (up to seven days) and Y male-producing sperm that swim faster but perish quicker (usually within three days). When Yin is ready to receive the Yang energy, she will open to allow only her chosen one entrance; he will simultaneously be embraced and beheaded. The original polar axis of the ova also determines the point at which the sperm will penetrate, and along which axis early cellular divisions will proceed, powered by prenatal Yuan

Qi. The nucleus from the male principle is taken inside where it blends with the nucleus of the egg. The spark is lit. A new dance begins.

It is friction that unites these opposing forces and that causes conflicts that will need to be worked out in life. The embrace of the Jing creates a vortex that will need to be ensouled to continue. As Water receives breath, the Lung–Kidney axis provides the force needed to keep life moving. If the embrace of the Jing creates the correct cosmic spark to attract an equal cosmic longing for materialization, an emergent lightning bolt from Heaven, full of lessons left over from previous incarnations, accepts this life vehicle and we have the three ingredients necessary to initiate life—Yin, Yang, and Po.

The formation of the Pei embryo implies that the heavenly inkling accepts the invitation of this Jing's embrace. The Po must be drawn to this particular platform of life, and take on its responsibility, associated with the Lung's ability to receive the breath of life, which is why the Conception Vessel's opening point is Lu 7 Lieque (Broken Sequence).

The life force is drawn inward, and the Three become One as the primordial Chong Mai. The first polar axis establishes the electric polarity by which the cell will split first into the Conception Vessel and its complementary Governing Meridian, and then by which all future meridians will proceed.

While science calls this process cleavage, the cell isn't whacked in two; it reproduces itself from within. Centrioles move to opposite sides of the cell where their polarity creates the traction to pull them apart. Enzymes break the DNA helix and the chromosomes split apart, giving each daughter cell 23 identical chromosomes. RNA replicates the inner process to complete the affair so each cell is identical. The Yin and Yang forces of radial and tangential energy, expansion, and contraction—one coiling inward, one expanding outward—divide again to four cells, giving rise to the Chong and Dai Mai (Belt Meridian) axis. The parental blueprints, read and interpreted by Chong Mai, create a three-dimensional reality consisting of up, down, front, and back. The constant tension between these two processes will create the appearance of separation and reunion for the rest of its life.

As this celestial body, propelled by Yuan Qi, proceeds down the fallopian tube over the next five days, it continues to divide into horizontal and vertical segments as it gives rise to the rest of the Eight Extraordinary Meridians that will direct various developmental stages after birth, and will then form a compact mass of 16 cells, named a morula (Latin for mulberry). On day six, a cavity of fluid forms in the center and we call it a blastocyst. Still occupying the same mass, it complexes into an inner cell mass that will form the embryo, outer cells that form into a trophoblast that will latch onto the endometrium, and a liquid-filled cavity, the blastocoele. This salty Jin fluid in the inner cavity, powered by San Jiao, will be responsible for nourishing the tremendous energy expenditure it will take to drive the embryo's duplicating process until the outer cell membrane is able to share in the mother's blood. The soul takes a drink of its inner ocean and ventures on.

Unless we are rooted in the Mysterious Mother herself, we do not have the power to intervene at this level. Chinese medical doctors can help prepare the palace by addressing the patterns of imbalance the patients exhibit, regulating the menstrual cycle, and improving Qi and Blood flow to the reproductive organs (E stim from UB 23–32) prior to implantation. Zigongxue and auricular ovary correspond to the ovaries; the Liver channel passes through the fallopian tubes; and the uterus can be impacted directly or indirectly with acupoints Sp 6 Sanyinjiao (Three Yin Intersection), Ll 4 Hegu (Joining Valley), St 29 Guilai (Return), St 30 Qichong (Surging Qi), Ren 4–7, UB 23 Shenshu (Kidney Transporter), UB 52 Zhishi (Will Chamber), UB 31–34, Ki 11–16, and auricular uterus. But we don't actively *cause* conception or implantation. We honor that these processes may be occurring while we address the patient's concerns. You may palpate the points of the Conception Vessel and Governing Vessel, looking for flaccid or stuck, gummy areas to needle. One of the best ways we can support our patients at this time is to calm the Shen, reduce anxiety, and open the chest with points such as Ht 7 Shenmen (Spirit Gate) or Pc 6 Neiguan (Inner Pass).

But we can also go back to our original question of where life originates. Taoist practitioners queried where the origin of Source Qi was located prior to Yin and Yang division, or where was the "mouth of Qi"? While it might be seen as a physical location like Lu 9 Taiyuan (Supreme Abyss), I think of it as an internal place where we are rooted in Heaven within and can touch these places in another. We could consider points such as Du 26 Renzhong (Water Trough) for the reception of Qi. St 9 Renying (Person's Welcome) welcomes our own humanity. St 25 Tianshu (Heaven's Pivot) is the source of the celestial polestar between Heaven and Earth. St 23 Taiyi (Supreme Unity) contains our heavenly true basic Qi; Ren 3 Zhongji (Central Pole) was described as the center of Heaven, like the body's north star around which the original movement of the Qi revolves; and Ren 19 Zigong (Purple Palace) calls to the place where the immortals dwell.

Ge Hong's Nine Flower technique, also known as Chong Mai's Nine Palace treatment, utilizes:

- Ki 21 Youmen (Hidden Gate) to enter the gate of the mystery
- Ki 23 Shenfeng (Spirit Seal) diffuses the Lung Qi to allow letting go, which will purify our vibration
- St 19 Burong (Not Contained), which can help support that which is not contained, like a child, when Earth can't consolidate its Qi
- Ki 19 Yindu (Yin's Metropolis), where distractions may be soothed and settled, and
- Ren 14 Jueque (Great Palace Gateway) allows us to survey the world around us and to feel comfortable in the environment we occupy; also where the sage baby strings the seven gold coins that represent the stars of the Big Dipper.

Together these points create an infinity symbol right at the junction where the dark, soft underbelly rises to meet the rib cage, like ocean waves lapping at the land that encases the spirit. This ritualistic needling sequence can cool the diaphragm and open Heart–Kidney communication to reinforce a healthy ascent up the Chong Mai, and can also help one call out their own hidden darkness in a blocked Chong Mai accessing infinity.

Implantation: entrance into the main chamber

In the depths of Yin, Yang begins to stir.

There is a lot going on during the process of implantation, and here receptivity is our superpower. The mother's Liver energies move to the Dai Mai to support Kidney Essence. As Water and Metal have combined, the Po soul will need to be banked by Earth in the lower Dan Tien, where all of the primary organ structures necessary for survival will be laid down during the first trimester. As we know, Earth initiates Tian Gui (heavenly Essence) production in the reverse generative cycle, and Earth upholds the embryo; thus, many formulae that encourage implantation and "prevent" miscarriage begin with a base of Qi and Blood tonics. After ovulation, the Heart has sent its Blood via the reverse cycle to the Liver.

The Pericardium must be capable of cooling the Blood, so Dan Shen may be employed prior to implantation.

Heart Blood goes to the Liver for storage, which is then delivered to the Dai Mai to support the Kidney Jing, and then to Zi Gong via Bao Lou. Wood is the dominant element during the first two months, and the status of the endometrium and the implanting embryo it will house depends on Liver Blood. When you press down on the deep position of the left Guan position, you should be able to feel a rise in the deep left Chi position, indicating that the Kidneys are receiving Liver Blood.

Kidney Yang increases Lung and Wei Qi activity at ovulation, and thereafter follows a complex response of immune modulation beneath the surface. Under the influence of progesterone, Yang stirs within the Yin endometrium, which undergoes a process called decidualization to enhance cyclic adenosine monophosphate (cAMP), an important biological messenger. The uterine lining now develops new vasculature, exhibits special mucus glands, and alters the expression of regulatory factors like cytokines, proteinases integrin, histocompatibility molecules, and white blood cells. All of this sophisticated Wei Qi activity is necessary for implantation. As the embryoblast communicates to the endometrium that it is looking for a home, it emits human chorionic gonadotropin (hCG) and responds to paracrine signals such as epidermal growth factor and leukemia inhibitory factor, like homing devices that prompt the surface epithelium to change configuration. The endometrium's gene expression must be modulated so it can signal back like a lighthouse that the lining is hospitable and the embryo can moor here. The internal Yang activity shifts—natural killer cells must be inactivated while cyclooxyrgenase 2, prostaglandins, cytokines, and growth factors must be regulated by the Liver and Spleen.

As the embryo docks, the trophoblast secretes enzymes (the same type of enzymes tumor cells emit) that digest the endometrium's extracellular matrix. As it buries deeper into the uterine stoma, like arms reaching toward its new home (according to the Nei Jing, *the Liver is delighted by orderly reaching*), the trophoblast cells divide into membranes that will become the chorion—the fetal portion of the placenta, the inner tree of life. More enzymes and signaling factors reconfigure the uterine vasculature, where maternal and fetal blood diffuse into the chorionic villi to allow the embryo to share in the pooled uterine blood that promises the fetus nutrients and oxygen.

All of the extra immune modulation is required because we have an invasion by an external factor here, a little Gui Po. Composed partly of self and partly of non-self, the embryonic invader has to be protected from our immune system because it meets all of the criteria for clean-up. But an intelligent immune system is able to differentiate that this one is meant to be here; it sends out cloaking molecules and settles down overactivity. About a week after ovulation, Wei Qi arrives at Ming Men and shifts the moving Qi of the Kidneys (which is also Chong Mai) forward to Zi Gong, where Kidney Yin and Liver Blood must be both sufficient and flowing smoothly to handle the immense Yang activity going on beneath the surface. The mother may experience spotting, bleeding, and some-times little uterine twinges during implantation. Most often, however, implan-tation goes unnoticed. Any interruption in blood flow can clot off the blood supply to the embryo; hence Dang Gui (angelica) and Chuan Xiong (cnidium) have historically been used to simultaneously tonify and invigorate the Blood to support implantation. Herbs like E Jiao (ass-hide gelatin) encourage the warm, sticky environment by which implantation succeeds. But we have to watch for too much stickiness; Damp Heat in the Lower Jiao must be avoided as it can be tricky to drain Dampness while upholding a fetus. Excess immune activity can be reduced with fish oil and Chai Hu Gui Zhi Gan Jiang Tang (Bupleurum, Cin-namon Twig and Ginger Decoction) with Tian Hua Fen (trichosanthis), Huang Qin (skullcap root), Mu Li (oyster shell), and Zhi Gan Cao (prepared licorice).

Many issues can interfere with implantation. The first two belong to the embryo: (1) either its Jing hasn't combined with a genetic sequence compatible for life, or (2) it isn't strong enough to propel the embryo with enough Yuan Qi to make it all the way from fertilization until it burrows into its uterine home to share in the mother's Blood supply. If it belongs to the former, we go back to preconception preparation. We can't modify its starting point. But along with certain cases of embryonic growth retardation, we can tonify the Kidneys and increase circulation to the uterus with Moxa over the Ba Liao points (UB 31–34).

Other implantation impediments belong to the mother, including uter-ine abnormalities, endometriosis or infections, hormonal disorders, chronic illnesses, and immunologic issues, which can be difficult to diagnose. We can utilize Sp 8 Diji (Earth Pivot) to invigorate the Xi-cleft point of the Spleen; St 36 Zusanli (Leg Three Miles) and Du 20 Baihui (Hundred Convergences) can help tonify and lift the Qi; and Pc 6 Neiguan (Inner Pass) can calm the Shen. But it's crucial to discern the status of her Blood-building organs, the Spleen, Liver, and Heart. Are they strong enough to support the embryo during the first trimester?

Is Chong Mai able to bank the Earth? Is her Heart and mind quiet enough to keep the emotions calm and refrain from heating the Blood? Autoimmune reactivity can also be a divergent issue of the second confluence Liver and Gallbladder, where Blood is the medium of holding, Ren 2 Qugu (Crooked Bone) is the lower confluent point and GB 1 Tongziliao (Pupil Crevice) the upper.

Early embryonic development

The embryo, or Pei, is described as a muddy substance composed by the combination of Yin and Yang. Throughout the first trimester, if growing adequately, it will continue emitting beta hCG, which should be doubling every two days. Upheld by its yellow satellite Spleen, the corpus luteum will be responsible for progesterone production for the next nine weeks until the placenta is mature and the main organ systems are laid down toward the end of the first trimester.

As our little Pei implants itself into the uterine lining, the quality of the pulse begins to undergo subtle changes. The mother's skin feels warmer to the touch as your fingers press in to meet the pulsing Blood, which takes on a more buoyant quality, becoming slippery, like a wave within a wave. The Heart and Kidney Yin pulses become more full and jubilant. However, as the embryo utilizes Liver Blood, the left Guan pulse, which should be full and taut but not wiry, will sink into the deep position, where, instead of moving distal toward the Cun to engender Heart Qi, it tucks in toward the deep Chi position to support Kidney Yin. This shows us just how crucial Liver Blood is to nourish the uterine lining and the developing embryo. Further, because Lung Qi will be descending more to support Kidney Qi, the right Cun pulse won't be diffusing to the surface as much, and instead will be reaching deeper. The right Guan may also show a discrepancy between the moderate and deep levels as they are trying to harmonize. All this is normal.

As the Conception Vessel is the first primal meridian to form, it follows that the first embryonic tissue to develop is said to be Po Men, the anus, followed by the mouth; as in all processes of renewal, release precedes intake. This creates an empty tube around which the flesh of the fetus forms. Our first level of priority is survival, which, after birth, will be governed by the Lung, Large Intestine, Stomach, and Spleen. After birth the initial tube from mouth to anus will allow the new being to breathe, eat, drink, absorb, and eliminate.

Concurrently, the central nervous system will begin to develop as a physical extension of life, generating electric currents as the Governing Meridian enlivens the Conception Meridian, and gives rise to the spinal column and nerves. The Yellow Emperor said in the *Ling Shu* that *after conception, the Jing is first composed. Then the Jing composes the brain and bone marrow.*

As our little embryo's rudimentary muddy substance is busy absorbing the basic heavenly organizing principles of life into the Eight Extraordinary Meridians, it also synchronizes the prenatal, fated constitutional factors like the genetic code, with environmental influences that will create the being's postnatal destiny. The *Su Wen* says, *eight in the mist become twelve in the distinct.* In another week or so, our Pei will begin the process of gastrulation, where the visibly undifferentiated substance will organize itself into three characteristically distinct cellular layers—endoderm, ectoderm and mesoderm—from which the twelve primary meridians will form.

Caring for the first month

While treatment strategies have been provided to prepare for implantation, we don't actively "treat" anything unless a process goes awry. Continue to address the mother's presenting patterns. Tonify what's deficient; resolve what's excess. Calm the Shen and encourage rest. Pc 6 Neiguan (Inner Pass) can and probably should be used during every treatment. *The Taishanshu states: In the first month it is called "flowing into the form." Food and drink must be the finest; the sour boiled dish must be thoroughly cooked. Do not eat acrid or rank foods. This is called "initial fixture."* Sour foods and herbs will help nourish the Liver and astringe its Blood. While we want to make sure the Lower Jiao has adequate Blood and Qi, now we are better advised to help lift and support the Earth. We can utilize points above the umbilicus like Ren 12 Zhongwan (Middle Epigastrium); we can strengthen the Spleen with UB 20 Pishu (Spleen's Hollow), and we can lift the Qi with Du 20 Baihui (Hundred Convergences). The gynecologist Huang Fu Mi recommends Ki 2 Rangu (Blazing Valley) to provide the fire to chisel the embryo into Sp 8 Diji (Earth Pivot), the major point for the uterus, which takes Earth into flight.

Try to avoid unnecessary acupuncture and moxibustion on the Liver channel. We can attend to the Liver by understanding and addressing its deeper functions. An inner story lies inside our Liver Blood, giving rise to our dreams, visions, and the way we perceive the world. Remember Xiang 相, mutual arising? As the Hun arise to the eyes to project the world, they bring with them the imagery and emotions of our conditioning. Outer events may activate the inner drama, and we respond not to what is, but what we are. I don't see the same tree you see. I see what a tree means to me. All of our views, the ones we like and the ones we don't like, will imprint their pattern on our creations. The first month is about softening the Liver; it's also about softening our viewpoints so the Hun can reach into the collective unconscious and allow new possibilities to arise.

A common herbal formula used during early pregnancy is Tai Shan Pan Shi San (Formula that Gives the Stability of Mount Tai), which provides stability, like Mount Tai. Composed of Ren Shen (ginseng), Huang Qi (astragalus), Bai Zhu (atractylodes), Shu Di Huang (rehmannia), Bai Shao (white peony), Chuan Xiong (cnidium), Dang Gui (angelica), Xu Duan (dipsacus), Huang Qin (skullcap root), Sha Ren (amomi), Nuo Dao Gen (glutinous rice), and Zhi Gan Cao (prepared licorice), it tonifies Qi and Blood, and prevents miscarriage with herbs that calm the fetus. It should, of course, be modified based on the patient's actual presentation.

Other herbs used during the first couple of months include Sang Ji Sheng (mulberry mistletoe), which is sometimes added to help nourish the Blood to support Jing. Xu Duan (dipsacus) is often used throughout pregnancy as it helps mobilize the hundred joints and activate the structure. Da Zao (Chinese date) tonifies the Spleen, the Blood, and calms the spirit. Huang Qin (skullcap root) helps to clear Heat that might contribute to restless fetus syndrome. Ai Ye (mugwort) warms the uterus to stop bleeding and pacifies the fetus, and E Jiao (ass-hide gelatin) nourishes the Blood. To ensure the Blood isn't overly congealed, move as you tonify. Make sure the Liver has adequate Blood and is not too hot or too cold. Wu Zhu Yu (evodia fruit) is the best herb to regulate the Liver and harmonize the Spleen and Stomach now. Liver Fire can exhaust Liver Blood in the first month; if the pulse is rapid, consider adding Mu Dan Pi (dried peony root bark). But watch out for Cold in the Liver, which causes Liver Blood stagnation. Fish oil capsules can nourish the Jing and mildly invigorate the Blood as well as support the developing fetal nervous system.

Throughout pregnancy it is advisable to avoid herbal purgatives, diaphoretics, and diuretics. We are also warned not to needle points designated "forbidden" during pregnancy; Sp 6 Sanyinjiao (Three Yin Intersection) and Ll 4 Hegu (Joining Valley) affect the uterus. But remember, acupuncture is meant to be *regulatory*. When the uterus is calm, these two points have the potential to agitate the uterus, but when the uterus is agitated and the woman is cramping, they may be the only points that are strong enough to shift the dynamic. Sp 4 Gongsun (Grandfather-Grandson) also has a relaxing effect on the uterus, and since it isn't contraindicated, try it first. If the woman is cramping, massage the auricular uterus point. If it becomes red or inflamed, use an ear seed.

GB 21 Jianjing (Shoulder Well) connects with the uterus while provoking a downward movement. Points like St 36 Zusanli (Leg Three Miles), GB 34 Yanglingquan (Yang Mound Spring), and Lv 3 Taichong (Great Surge) have a strong effect on the Qi, so cautionary use is advised. Of course, when we pay attention to the patient's signs, symptoms, tongue, and pulse, we might be able to use them. Check the pulse before and immediately after you needle any of these relatively contraindicated points. See if the symptoms or pulse quality normalizes. If you don't feel confident in your pulse-taking skills and have any hesitancy, it is best to go back to the rules and don't use these points at all. Needling the Heart and Small Intestine meridians is discouraged throughout gestation.

Risk of pregnancy loss and miscarriage prevention

During the first month, the woman may only just be discovering she is newly pregnant. Some women miscarry without even missing a period. They may feel like they were pregnant and have some symptoms of early pregnancy, but their periods arrive. Some may have periods that are heavier than normal and contain some fibrous tissue. Some may have delayed periods or have a verified pregnancy (with + beta hCG), only to be told they had a "chemical" pregnancy where the test was positive but no conceptus is present on ultrasound. They were pregnant, but it didn't survive long enough to grow and continue. Equally distasteful medical diagnostic terms are "blighted ovum" and "spontaneous abortion." Neither takes into account the emotional toll a woman who has been trying to conceive experiences. She has lost a hoped-for child, and her Heart will need to be addressed.

The majority of miscarriages will occur during the first trimester, when the major organ systems are developing, although complicated issues can result in losses any time throughout pregnancy. The later the loss, the more physically and emotionally devastating it will be. But do not discount the toll earlier losses will take on her body, mind, and spirit. Any time a pregnancy ends prematurely without delivering a live child, it will take a while for the mother's system to recalibrate.

Some of the terms used to refer to pregnancy loss and miscarriage are:

- An Chan: miscarriage in the first month.
- Duo Tai: miscarriage in the first trimester.
- Tai Lou: threatened miscarriage—vaginal Bleeding during pregnancy.
- Tai Dong Bu An: restless fetus—vaginal bleeding, backache, abdominal pain, and bearing-down sensation.
- An Tai: fetal leakage—calm the fetus.
- Shou Tai: prolong the life of the fetus—Jing is deficient.
- Bao Tai: protect the fetus when Jing, Qi, and Blood deficiency are present.
- Yang Tai: nurture the fetus—when Yin is deficient.
- Shi Tai: treat the fetus—bleeding needs to be staunched immediately.
- Ban Shan: refers to miscarriages after the first trimester.

Immunologic and autoimmune implantation failures may show up with immune markers that indicate the body isn't accepting the implanting embryo, or that the mother's immune cells are actively rejecting it. Reproductive specialists can do complex endometrial biopsies and test for the presence of the necessary T cell-blocking antibody, or elevated levels of natural killer cells, antinuclear antibodies, cytotoxic lymphocytes, and antiphospholipid, lupus anticoagulant, and anticardiolipin antibodies. Whatever the marker, they will always show up with a pattern of imbalance. A high percentage of immunoregulatory defects manifest with patterns of Liver Blood deficiency and Spleen Qi vacuity, which then allows latent Heat to escape into the Blood and destroy the tissue. It can also begin with an underlying Qi, Blood, Yin, or Yang deficiency compounded by patterns of Blood stasis, Heat, Dampness, Damp Heat, Toxic Heat, or any combination.

Maternal immune reactions are not the only causes of miscarriage; they can also result from weak Jing, infections that cause Damp Heat, Wind-Heat, or Wind-Cold that may produce fevers, and Blood toxins and accidents that may disrupt the Bao Mai. The pulse can give us some clues.

A healthy pregnancy pulse is strong and slippery. During the first month of pregnancy, the deep Liver pulse will become stronger than the other positions. This is normal and natural, as the Liver energies should be coursing deeply to support the pregnancy. If they remain wiry and superficial, the Liver Blood may not support implantation. A pregnancy may be interrupted with no signs or symptoms at all. The pulse may lose its slippery quality, although this is not diagnostic by itself, as the slippery quality may come and go. If it is accompanied by a choppy feel, make sure the Blood is sufficient and moving adequately. Address tightness in the pulse, freeing up the Qi mechanism to support the pregnancy. Floating Kidney Yang pulses indicate that the Wei Qi is trying to rid itself of the pregnancy. When they are weak and floating, make sure to use astringent herbs to help stop the leakage. When both left and right pulses are weak and tight, it may indicate uterine Cold is displacing the Yang Qi, which then rises up. Rou Gui (cinnamon bark), Gan Jiang (ginger), and Fu Zi (wolfsbane) can root the Yang Qi, at which time Fu Zi should be discontinued.

Signs and symptoms of a potential interrupted pregnancy include:

- Low back pain—indicating Kidney Essence vacuity and/or Liver Yin vacuity. Warming the low back can help, although avoid extreme heat. Use UB 23 Shenshu (Kidney Transporter), UB 52 Zhishi (Will Chamber), and Ren 4 Guanyuan (Origin Pass).
- Cramping—first address the pattern that is causing the cramping. If it is severe and tight, think Cold; pressure/bloating/wringing indicate Qi stagnation; stabbing suggests Blood stasis; and downbearing may indicate Spleen Qi vacuity. Treat the pattern and try points that relax—Sp 4 Gongsun (Grandfather-Grandson), Pc 6 Neiguan (Inner Pass), Ht 7 Shenmen (Spirit Gate); check ear uterus point for reactivity and needle if positive. If the above isn't successful, add Sp 6 Sanyinjiao (Three Yin Intersection) and recheck the pulse. If the uterus is still reactive, add Ll 4 Hegu (Joining Valley).
- Bleeding—it is estimated that bleeding occurs in approximately 20% of pregnancies. TCM causes of bleeding include trauma, Spleen Qi, and/or Kidney Qi vacuity (may be pinkish or watery); Blood stasis (darker in color); or Heat (bright red). The herbal formula E Jiao Ai Tang (Ass-Hide Gelatin and Mugwort Formula) helps to nourish and invigorate Blood and contain leakage. E Jiao (ass-hide gelatin) is usually the first herb to address spotting and bleeding. Vegetarians can use Yi Mu Cao (Chinese motherwort), but it is slower to curtail the Bleeding. When building Blood, we also need to invigorate to prevent Blood stasis.

Each of these symptoms by themselves doesn't necessarily need to cause grave concern. When all three are present, however, the outlook is poorer. Where maternal and fetal circulation mingle, the Blood can congeal, showing subchorionic hematoma via ultrasound. Blood stasis is often the culprit; often we need to invigorate Yang to move the Blood. Sp 10 Xuehai (Sea of Blood), UB 17 Geshu (Diaphragm's Hollow), and Moxa to Ren 4 Guanyuan (Origin Pass) and Du 4 Mingmen (Gate of Destiny) can help. Blood stasis is often the first sign of immune reactivity as the body clots off the blood supply to starve the invading embryo. If blood-clotting laboratory abnormalities are found, the obstetrician may prescribe a drug like heparin, which moves the Blood but depletes Kidney Yang. We can address these issues safely by incorporating herbs with a Blood-invigorating effect such as Dang Gui (angelica), Pu Huang (typhae pollen), Yi Mu Cao (Chinese motherwort) or Ai Ye (mugwort) to the appropriate herbal formula to address the pattern, or modify Tai Shan Pan Shi Tang (Formula that Gives the Stability of Mount Tai). Charred Jing Jie (schizonepeta) is also effective to stop bleeding.

Uterine Blood stasis is often due to Cold; the pulse will tend to be slower and tight. Herbs that cool the Blood can also cool Yang and potentially the creative force. Kidney Yang is also required to move the Blood. We have to have enough warmth to create the child, but not too much to Heat the Blood.

Maternal taxation may cause, accompany, or exacerbate other patterns, depleting Qi and Blood. When extreme fatigue accompanies any pattern, consider St 36 Zusanli (Leg Three Miles), and Du 20 Baihui (Hundred Convergences) along with Ki 16 Huangshu (Vitals Transporter) and Tituo to help lift and hold. Bu Zhong Yi Qi Tang (Tonify the Middle and Augment the Qi Decoction) is a great choice to ascend the Qi. Sheng Ma (cimicifuga) and Chai Hu (bupleurum) lift Spleen energies, but can be drying. When Qi is deficient, Blood will also suffer. Leakage of Blood is likely, and the pulse will often float to the surface. Huang Qi helps support Yuan Qi, and astringents like Gou Qi Zi (Chinese wolfberry), Suan Zao Ren (sour jujube), Bai Shao (white peony), Fu Pen Zi (Chinese raspberry), and Wu Wei Zi (schisandra berry) can help astringe Jing and thicken the Blood to prevent leakage. Xu Duan (dipsacus) helps to mesh everything together. Sang Ji Sheng (mulberry mistletoe) is the major herb to address Yin, and Tu Si Zi (cuscuta) will help astringe and nourish Yang.

When the Yin is weak, especially in women in their later reproductive years, spotting often begins in the evenings. In this case we will need to nourish the Yin to hold onto the Yang. Our formulations will need to include Yin tonics like Han Lian Cao (eclipta) and Nu Zhen Zi (privet fruit) as well as Huang Qin (skullcap root) when Heat is present (rapid pulse, red tongue, feelings of subjective heat). Shan Yao (Chinese yam) helps the Spleen bank the Blood and promotes progesterone production; Mai Men Dong (ophiopogan) and Tian Men Dong (asparagus tuber) should be added in when Lung and Stomach Yin are also deficient. Tonify the Kidneys with Ki 3 Taixi (Supreme Stream), Ki 7 Fuliu (Returning Current), UB 23 Shenshu (Kidney Transporter), and Ren 4 Guanyuan (Origin Pass).

Lila was referred by a midwife when she was in process of her fifth miscarriage. I had never seen her before. She arrived knotted up and pale, with shoulder pain and severe uterine cramping. She was starting to spot, but the blood was light in amount and brown in color. Each of her previous miscarriages started this same way, around six weeks into the pregnancy. Her pulse was wiry in the left Guan position, and choppy and weak in the Chi position. Her Blood and Qi needed to move! Before I had a chance to (over) think, I needed the four gates (Ll 4 (Joining Valley) and Lv 3 (Great Surge)), Sp 6 Sanyinjiao (Three Yin Intersection), Sp 10 Xuehai (Sea of Blood), and Ashi points around GB 21 Jianjing (Shoulder Well). Her color came back and her pulses normalized. When her cramps subsided, I removed Ll 4 (Joining Valley) and the shoulder points, and gave her some Dang Gui and Chuan Xiong tea to drink. While she still needed some Qi and Blood invigorating during the next two months, her pregnancy proceeded with no other concerns. She gave birth at home.

Ectopic pregnancy

Ectopic means the pregnancy has occurred outside the uterus, 90% of which occur within the fallopian tubes. Women often have a history of pelvic inflammatory disease (PID) or previous ectopic pregnancies, both of which can cause scar tissue to develop. When a woman has this history, treatments invigorate the fallopian tubes by needling (often with E stim) lower abdominal points such as Zi Gong, St 28 Shuidao (Water Passage), St 29 Guilai (Return), and Ki 14 Siman (Four Fullness). Or open the Dai Mai with GB 41 Zulinqi (Foot Governor of Tears), along with GB 26 Daimai (Girdle Vessel), GB 27 Wushu (Five Pivots), and/or GB 28 Weidao (Linking Path). Massage the abdomen deeply with castor oil and essential oils that move the Blood, like Ru Xiang (frankincense). Needle auricular adnexa/pelvic cavity points if reactive to massage.

When the muddy substance of the embryo moves down the oviduct, it can get "stuck" if the cilia aren't moving adequately (raw Huang Qi (astragalus) helps with this). It may be caused by Lung Qi deficiency, which, along with Kidney Yang, shuttles the egg into the fallopian tube, which crosses the Liver channel, but is under the domain of the Gallbladder. If this transit is interrupted, classic signs and symptoms include bleeding and abdominal pain, which may be crampy, dull, or sharp. Some women are asymptomatic, however. Western diagnosis is via blood tests and ultrasound, but we can palpate the Chi pulses that tend to be slippery, tight, choppy, or wiry. The sublingual veins may also be blue. In addition to underlying patterns of Qi deficiency, patterns include Cold in the Liver/Gallbladder, Heat in the Lung, Damp Heat, Phlegm, and Stomach Fire. If the tube ruptures, severe bleeding may occur, which may lead to shock. An ectopic pregnancy cannot be saved, so we don't try to employ the methods to prevent miscarriage. We may, however, attempt to facilitate its passing.

When an embryo is stuck in the oviduct or has died in utero, it is no longer with soul; we may utilize the above points, along with Sp 6 Sanyinjiao (Three Yin Intersection), Sp 10 Xuehai (Sea of Blood), LI 4 Hegu (Joining Valley), and GB 21 Jianjing (Shoulder Well). If the tube hasn't ruptured, we may also be more liberal in our use of Blood movers. A formula to assist the body to resolve ectopic pregnancies utilizes 24 grams of Ji Xue Teng (spatholobus); 15 grams each of E Zhu (curcuma rhizome), San Leng (sparganium), and Wang Bu Liu Xing (vaccaria); 12 grams of Bai Zhu (atractylodes); and 9 grams of Zhi Ke (bitter orange). Other approaches include Da Huang (rhubarb root) to help purge the bowels, Tan Xiang (sandalwood), and Mu Xiang (aucklandia) to open the diaphragm.

Surgery may be required and the individual may lose a fallopian tube (still treat the other one, though, as pregnancy is still possible). Post-surgical treatment might include Yunnan White Herbal Medicine, Dan Shen Yin (Salvia Decoction), Yi Mu Cao (Chinese motherwort), or Tao Ren (peach kernel). After rupture or surgery, we want to reduce the likelihood of scar tissue. Zhi Ke (bitter orange) helps open the diaphragm to help move Blood. Along with UB 17 Geshu (Diaphragm's Hollow), as you open the diaphragm, you bring the Kidney Qi to the Heart so that the Heart can resolve the stagnation. Sp 21 Dabao (Great Embracement) can assist; Bai Zhu (atractylodes) will help build the Blood and ascend; and Yi Mu Cao (Chinese motherwort) and Ji Xue Teng (spatholobus)) will help build back Blood.

Emotional care of pregnancy loss

Regarding the soul, Po has begun manifesting in this existence, but that does not mean that its curriculum included being birthed and growing up. It may have intended to experience a beating heart, or being held in the mother's Blood, but not to accept the breath of Life. Pregnancies that do not come to term are one of the most challenging issues a woman may go through. Life has been interrupted, which is upsetting to the body, mind, spirit, hormones, and plans for one's life.

The sudden presence or emergence of fear may signal a problem. Fear causes the Qi to descend, which increases the likelihood of loss. Those who have had previous pregnancy losses, however, will tend to be more anxious. Calm the Shen and lift the Qi so the Heart–Kidney axis doesn't separate. It rarely helps to advise them not to be fearful after a previous pregnancy loss. This can cause latency to develop as they try to suppress the fear. Fear belongs to the Kidneys, and suppression to the Liver. Allow them to be sad and give voice to their fear so it can lose its power. Fear that one's child might be threatened is a natural part of parenting. In the meantime, you may reassure them that each pregnancy is unique, and they are in a different place now.

If attempts to forestall miscarriage are unsuccessful, encourage the mother to remain in bed while bleeding. While you can help expel the contents (as above), do not attempt to arrest bleeding if any fetal tissue remains. Bone marrow soup can be very nourishing, and when she is ready, Qi and Blood tonics, like Gui Pi Tang (Restoring the Spleen Decoction) that also nourish the Heart, can be helpful. Please do not offer platitudes; you do not know what it feels like for her, and nor do you know that her child is in a better place. Allow the space for her to express her sorrow without needing to fix it for her.

When the acute stage of mourning is over, some exercises that may be helpful include:

- Bury the residual contents of the pregnancy and plant a tree, flower, or bush over it.
- Journal or write a letter to the soul of their unborn child to express their feelings and any guilt they may have experienced for doing something "wrong."
- Light a candle for the child and say a prayer to or for it, together or alone.

MOTHERS' GUIDELINES FOR THE FIRST MONTH

Nutrition

During the first month, continue to strengthen your Spleen with the dietary guidelines given for preconception preparation. Then add in some sour and tart foods. These can include citrus and tart fruits, fermented and pickled foods. If you aren't gluten sensitive, allow yourself to eat glutinous whole grains. Barley is great to hydrate and support the Spleen. Root vegetables and baked beets, chicken, and bone broth will also help support the developing embryo. Fish and fish oil will be helpful for Blood flow and development of the nervous system.

Avoid highly refined foods, hot spicy foods, heavy, large meals, and anything with trans fats like margarine, and reduce or eliminate alcohol and all intoxicants. Avoid cold foods like ice, popsicles, and ice cream.

Unnecessary prescription and non-prescription drugs should be reduced, in consultation with your obstetrician, of course.

Drink peppermint or ginger tea, especially if you are feeling any digestive upset.

Lifestyle

Avoid getting overly heated or too cold. Free up and move your energy, but be careful not to overdo it, physically or mentally. Reduce strenuous exercise as the Liver also nourishes the sinews. Avoid heavy lifting. Excessive exercise can shunt the uterine Blood into the musculature. Be around animals, nature, and new life forms. Take a walk in the zoo. Make love freely. Do the things that move your soul. Surround yourself with things you find pleasant and valuable. It's important to bathe your body and mind with feelings of appreciation. The being within you is starting to share your Blood, which contains the imprint of your thoughts and feelings. It is extremely important to avoid stress—not only for your own health, but also the future health of your child. Stress hormones impact which parts of the fetal brain—forebrain or hindbrain—receive more developmental attention, setting them up for how they will tend to respond to stress for the rest of their lives.

Because the Liver will be nourishing the developing embryo, and the Liver also regulates and smooths emotions, it is important to deal with any emotional reactivity, especially anger. Repression, however, will just bottle it up inside and negatively impact both of you. When you feel angry, move the energy out of your body. Go for a walk. Release anger and resentment—use journaling or letter burning to bring these feelings out to release tension. Scream out loud or punch a pillow. Resolve feelings of frustration with forgiveness of self or others whenever possible, as stagnated emotion can inhibit the Qi mechanism. Laughter can lift the heaviness of all ailments, so watch a funny movie or call a friend whose sense of humor brings you to tears, to release any stuck internal feelings.

Therapeutic exercises

- Consider keeping a dream journal for your child, and keep your imagination active. Your own dreams and visions of your child are best served by remaining completely open and accepting. You can massage your Liver meridian, from the web between the second and third toes up to the groin, massaging the area over the lower belly and womb, and massaging up toward the rib cage, just below the nipples.
- Breathe deeply and relax—circulating the breath immediately drops stress levels, initiating the relaxation response and setting the stage for meditation. If you haven't gotten used to breathing into your lower abdomen yet, keep practicing! Deepen your breath, allowing your belly to expand as you bring your awareness to your pelvis. Feel a channel from your heart to your womb, and allow the energies between the two to merge. Expand this connection to your whole body and mind.
- Eye exercises—the liver is related to vision, so it is important to exercise the eyes to clear out stuck memories. Lying on the ground, look up, look down, to the right, to the left, and make big circles in each direction. Start with your eyes closed, and then do it with your eyes open, not focusing on objects, just scanning. This exercise repeated daily can help reprogram thoughts, calm the nervous system, and improve vision.
- Bring your inner awareness to the uterus while your fingers rest on the skin over your uterus. As you inhale, lift your breath, your awareness, and your fingertips to your heart. With your fingertips over your sternum, exhale as you open up your arms in a circle, first in front and then to the side, as if you are blessing a crowd. Return your fingers to over your womb and begin again.

Self-inquiry exercises

Because the Liver governs our dreams and desires, it is important to allow yourself to dream and desire, but not excessively. Desires that exceed the Liver Blood's ability to manifest them can have a detrimental effect on the pregnancy. Dream for your baby, but don't outline too definitively about how it should appear. See if you can open your mind to its developing potential without imposing your own image of what it should look like.

Here are some issues to consider to strengthen the Liver and dislodge stuck energies:

- Where is my Life Blood going—is it available to nourish me and a new life?
- Am I caring for other life endeavors at the expense of my own resources?
- Are there any plans that need to be instituted in my life?
- In what areas of my life do I need to make a change or a decision?
- Are there any aspects of my life that I have been trying to force that cause inner stress?
- What views do I hold that don't really work for me or anyone else any more?
- Do I have any unfulfilled desires I can let go?
- Are there any areas in life where I am meeting resistance?
- What issues do I need to accept and let be?
- Any place I am lacking compassion—for myself or others?
- What areas have presented a barrier despite my best efforts?
- What are my greatest dreams, visions, or aspirations?
- When has resistance, frustration, or anger prevented the fulfillment of my dreams or goals?
- What resentments do I still carry that I now have the possibility to release?
- What provides me with the greatest hope?

CHAPTER 6

Gallbladder: Lunar Month Two

Weeks 4–8

Days 29–56

> As the Master Carpenter carves the Unhewn,
> the Tao begins to take shape.

For any new endeavor to continue, what began as a hazy dream must begin to define itself in order to proceed to the next developmental stage. The second phase of the soul's incarnation correlates with infancy, where a distinct entity exists in this dimension, but because it has yet to be defined by this world, it remains consciously unaware of its separate existence. The Yang aspect of Wood provides the definition whereby we become one thing and not another, later giving rise to the faculty of decisiveness.

During the first month, the process of fertilization produced the Essence-rich Gao, undifferentiated fatty tissue, prior to any visible discernible stages of embryological organizational structure. Conception energetics supported by the Liver allowed the embryo to burrow into the endometrial lining and begin to share in the mother's Blood. Now that nourishment has been established, the Gallbladder's Yang activity will help support the Governing Meridian as this pasty substance begins to bulge into a fleshy swelling with form and substance. During the second lunar month of pregnancy, the inkling of materialization begins to gel into a more specific shape, where internal boundaries are formed as the Gallbladder composes mesenteric membranes from the Jing in the Bao's lining.

The *Huai Nan Zi* says, *In the second month, a corporeal mass develops.* A little refresher on Gallbladder energetics might help to understand the process that is about to occur.

> The universe is within, where the sun and moon
> rise and set within the cavern of your own Heart,
> somewhere around GB 24 Riyue (Sun and Moon).

The simple character for Gallbladder, Dan 胆, is composed of the flesh radical with the sun rising at dawn indicating the ability to rise up and burst forth with clarity. A more complex character 膽 shows a person bent in hesitancy over a dangerous cliff. In the presence of a threat, a decision must be made to choose the right way. Embodying the strength of Shao Yang, the Gallbladder has the power to break through barriers and open new possibilities with calm and anchored clarity, directing the appropriate way.

The Gallbladder is a bowel, but also holds pure precious Essence (bile, a thick Ye fluid to which Marrow belongs), making it a curious organ, like the uterus. Fu organs descend from Heaven and empty themselves; Essences, however, must rise up to communicate with Heaven. The Gallbladder, like its zigzagging trajectory, deals with paradox, fluctuations, and inconsistencies between up and down, in and out, left and right. Pure, clear, and exact, Qing describes the blue-green color of the ocean depths, bile, and the power of the dragon-like emergence of spring. Because it links with the Eight Extraordinary Vessels, it can tap into our constitution and is the only organ to wrap the genitals. Controlling both the Marrow and bones, it transports information to and from the brain. Later in life these might be habituated, rigid-holding patterns that we've been able to ignore because we lack the courage to step into what is required to change our lives.

In the Han dynasty, the Gallbladder was associated with fear. As the Yang aspect of Wood, it can express that which its mother, Water, may be unable to—the courage to confront one's fears. The strength of the Gallbladder can overcome the contraction of fear, hesitancy, and holding back, helping us to pierce through and rise above. Indecision carries the paralyzing discomfort of fear that we may make the wrong move. When prolonged, this toxic state gnaws away at the Jing. Jing holds our latency; Jing holds our fears. A healthy, strong

Gallbladder can help us move past fear of change, fear of Wind, and break out of the peril of our stagnant holding patterns. It can help us reduce the burden we've placed on our lives—physical, mental, emotional, or spiritual fixated points of view.

Awakening all transformations, the eleven organs go to the Gallbladder for decisions. The Gallbladder, whose I Ching hexagram is Return ䷗, consists of one Yang—arising under five Yins:

> Yin is quietude, yang is movement;
> when quietude reaches its consummation, it gives rise to movement.
> It is this point of movement that is the mysterious pass.

> —*Li Dao Chun's Zhong He Ji (The Book of Balance and Harmony)*

The Yin Liver stores, and when it reaches its zenith, the Gallbladder, which relates to reincarnation, can help release stuck fears and areas that are stagnant because we fear change. The Gallbladder provides the ability to be calm, to wait for the correct moment when the Essences of Heaven rise up and present a new possibility. The Gallbladder links Water with Fire, Jing with Shen, and Ministerial Fire with Sovereign Fire, providing the Yang to help us evolve toward our destiny.

Embryo development

Our embryo, saturated with Jing, has reached the peak of Wood's Yin potential. The Gao must be transformed, and there can be no hesitancy. Precision, exactness, and strength set the stage, and development takes off to establish spatial cavities. The Conception Vessel and Governing Vessel have synthesized into the being's own Yuan Qi, and the Dai Mai, closely associated with the Gallbladder, now becomes active. The Conception Vessel, Governing Vessel, and Chong Mai provide a two-dimensional vertical structure, and the Dai Mai provides the horizontal weave through which the Bao Mai wrap into the Huang membranes, establishing the internal latticework for the evolving structure of the soul to follow.

The *Lun Heng* says the human form is created by a solidification of Qi. Sun Si Miao says the embryo weaves itself into a knot. Now the Yang movement of the essential Qi will direct the expansion of a more complex form, and the trinity of development reappears. Three weeks after conception, through a Gallbladder-directed process called gastrulation, the blastula rearranges itself spatially, spinning into three layers, which will become the basis of every single cell in the body:

- Endoderm takes on the function of the Conception Vessel and nutritive Qi, becoming the endothelium of the gastrointestinal system and the urogenital systems—the pancreas and liver.
- Ectoderm takes on the function of Governing Vessel and defensive Qi, becoming the nervous system and body surface—skin, hair and nails.
- Mesoderm, associated with Chong Mai and Source Qi, becomes the heart, blood vessels, kidneys, spleen, connective tissues, and bones.

The Two become Three. Three weeks after conception, a primitive streak in the midline of the embryo allows the embryo to fold to form what will become the three burners. The ectoderm will fold into a neural tube by a process called neurulation, which will become the nervous system. The Pei has its own Essences now. Yuan Qi disseminates via Du Mai, which elongates the spine of the fetus. Du Mai distributes to the back Shu points of the Bladder, which will be imprinted with Ming when San Jiao takes over in the fourth month. The brain, spinal cord, and eye lens begins to form. Our little Pei is going through the same primordial evolutionary stages that have brought it to being and make it virtually undistinguishable from a reptilian embryo. Yet soon, those little nerves and eyes will begin absorbing the imprints of the mother, through its earliest educational setting.

Caring for the second month

During this dynamic time, when both the Governing and Gallbladder networks become active, we attempt to keep things stable and in place, with consolidation our goal. As form is beginning to take shape, the mother's Jing is given to create the initial tissues. Her Earth element is busy banking the process of Life, which may tax her Spleen and leave her fatigued. Her Liver is trying to get the Blood to be stored in the Kidney to support the pregnancy, and her Gallbladder takes the thick Ye fluid to support and activate the Jing.

As Liver dominance passes into its Wood Yang phase, the mother may experience sudden and strange cravings. She may also experience joint pains, anxiety, and alternating Heat and Cold. She should avoid extremes—in conditions, emotions, and activities. Strong scents can even overly arouse the Wei Qi at this time; we don't want the Yang to become too active on the surface. During this time, the Lung Qi is descending. The Liver has been sending its Blood to the uterus. The Gallbladder transports the Ye to support the Jing, and the Pericardium calms the spirit by bringing the Heart to the Kidneys. All of this downward movement must be countered by the Spleen, which needs to ascend to keep the fetus from prolapsing. While many obstetricians want to move Blood down, that would be mimicking the actions of Cold, which is not welcome now. We want to bring the energy in and up, astringe leakages, harmonize Shao Yang, and tonify Kidney Yin and Yang without being too moving or too warming.

In the second month, some of the rules change. *The Taichanshu* says: *The dwelling place must be still.* As we've moved from a Yin to a Yang meridian, there are now more prohibitions. While women are free to enjoy sex during the first month, they should avoid sex now. While sour tastes are still encouraged, fermented foods are not, since they can restrict the Gallbladder's ability to nourish the Heart and Kidney. During the second month, avoid needling the Gallbladder channel, but do bring in Liver points to harmonize Qi. We can also use points on the Yang Wei Mai. If a Dai Mai pulse appears in the second month (a vibrating or moving in the Guan position), it indicates unsteadiness. The Liver pulse should be tight in the first trimester, as it needs to give its Blood to the Kidney, but shouldn't be overly tight, which would indicate Cold in the Liver or Gallbladder. Emotional holding may be behind this—encourage the release of stuck emotions with Lv 5 Ligou (Woodworm Canal). Wiry or tight Spleen or Stomach pulses may also indicate Cold.

The principle herbs that might be added during the second month include Huang Lian (coptis), Ai Ye (mugwort), Qian Shi (euryales), and Tu Si Zi (cuscuta). Xu Duan (dipsacus)—a hundred joints can help knit together any weakness, especially when there's joint pain or weakness. In addition to addressing underlying patterns, our treatment principles are to consolidate—warm what's cool; cool what's warm; harmonize any counterflow; and astringe what's leaking. While we will do the same with acupuncture and Moxa, we can also include Ht 6 Yinxi (Yin Cleft), a recommended point during the second lunar month. Further, the master point for Gao is Ren 15 Jiuwei (Turtledove Tail), which can help provide the Yin substance that will wrap around the organs. Huang membrane's master point is Ren 6 Qihai (Sea of Qi), which can strengthen the ability for substances to move in and out through the wrappings. We can use UB 43 Gaohuangshu (Vital Region Shu) to release scapular heat, perhaps shunted over from UB 14 Jueyinshu (Absolute Yin). And the governing point for the Bao is Sp 8 Diji (Earth Pivot).

The Lungs provide Qi to the lower burner, move the Blood and protect the Gao membrane. The Lung Qi goes to the Kidney, which siphons Qi to the center to support fetal development. The Lung pulse should not be rapid; if it is clear, Heat from the Lungs (Lu 10 Yuji (Fish Border)). Further, if Kidney Yin is deficient, Lung Yin may also become deficient—consider Mai Men Dong Tang (Ophiopogonis Decoction). This is more common in older maternal age. Sometimes the process of living exhausts the Yang Qi, Lungs included. Invigorating the life force is important here. When Lung Qi weakens, respiratory infections are more common. Add raw Huang Qi (astragalus) to whatever other formula they are on (Bu Zhong Yi Qi Tang (Tonify the Middle and Augment the Qi Decoction) is also a great formula to tonify Lung Qi).

We have moved from a pasty lump into the complex distribution of Qi between different levels. But we haven't lost the Gao; it remains as the rudimentary substance between Tao and self, now with membranes of division. The anonymous 14th-century author of *The Cloud of Unknowing* says that because humans feel and know that they are, they remain a "lump" of self, tormented with a sense of being separate that makes them nearly mad with sorrow. As soon as we differentiate into substance with complexity, an inside and an outside, harmony between levels may be lost. Chinese medicine refers to this as disharmony between the nutritive and defensive levels. Restoring Ying/Wei harmony is a common treatment principle, but what does it actually mean? In the second month of pregnancy we may need to address counterflow, restore flow, and calm down any overactivity manifesting through the mother. But later in life, this particular disharmony often stems from one's interior life being at odds with their exterior life. They may lack harmony between what nourishes their soul and the face they show the world, and may expend their Qi defending a false persona. This can only produce internal conflict, which will, of course, be passed on to their creations.

Developmental stalls

When a woman's obstetrician tells her that growth seems to have been arrested or the embryo is measuring smaller than expected on ultrasound, it doesn't necessarily mean the pregnancy is over. Intrauterine growth retardation (IUGR) just means that the embryo is measuring small for gestational age. It could be due to reduced Qi and Blood flowing to the uterus, which is often due to overexertion, which exhausts them. While tonifying Qi, Blood, Yin, and Yang is crucial, our treatment principles need to include returning that Qi and Blood to the center. The mother should be able to breathe into and focus her attention on the uterus, while lifting up the pelvic floor. While all of the substances must be contained, this is also the time when Yang must activate them. We can needle or Moxa the Ba Liao points (UB 31–34).

- Add St 36 Zusanli (Leg Three Miles) and UB 17 Geshu (Diaphragm's Hollow) to tonify and invigorate the Blood.
- For Liver Blood deficiency, include UB 18 Ganshu (Liver Shu), UB 20 Pishu (Spleen's Hollow), and Lv 8 Ququan (Spring at the Bend).
- For Heart Blood deficiency, include Pc 4 Ximen (Xi Cleft Gate), UB 20 Pishu (Spleen's Hollow), UB 17 Geshu (Diaphragm's Hollow), and St 36 Zusanli (Leg Three Miles).
- For Spleen Yang deficiency, include St 36 Zusanli (Leg Three Miles) and UB 20 Pishu (Spleen's Hollow).
- For Kidney Yang deficiency, include UB 23 Shenshu (Kidney Transporter), UB 52 Zhishi (Will Chamber), Ren 4 Guanyuan (Origin Pass), and Du 4 Mingmen (Gate of Destiny) with Moxa.

Molar pregnancies

A molar pregnancy, also called a hytadidiform mole, is a rare disorder during early pregnancy where the trophoblast cells that usually develop into the placenta grow out of control. A molar pregnancy starts out like any other pregnancy, but often develops symptoms like pelvic pressure or pain, vaginal passage of blood, or grape-like cysts, and severe nausea and vomiting, as grape-like clusters grow rapidly, like uncontrolled Gao, which is Yin; hCG rises dramatically. The uterus may grow much more quickly than usual, and the process can devolve into causing hypertension and preeclampsia. This is caused when two sperm get in to fertilize an egg—either the chromosomal material of the mother doesn't participate in replication or the father's genetic material replicates. Here we can ask what might cause the Yin to be unable to regulate the Yang, which overrides these boundaries? The egg's Wei Qi opens and closes its boundaries, like pores, to allow one sperm in. Perhaps there is too much Heat in the lower burner. Perhaps she is Yin-deficient or her Lungs are unable to communicate with the Kidneys. Whatever the case, it results in excess Yang.

Chinese medicine views this as the Gao Huang being unable to contain and astringe. Excess Yang during this time can override the Gallbladder's ability to compartmentalize, and it basically ferments, like too much yeast in dough, causing it to leak out of its container. Molar pregnancies can also lead to a rare type of cancer. While this pregnancy can't be saved, we can help clear Heat and Damp Heat in the Lower Jiao, and strengthen the Lung to reduce its likelihood (1 in 100) of happening again.

Anemia

Anemia describes a certain thinness of the Blood caused by iron deficiency; without adequate iron, the body can't produce enough hemoglobin, the oxygen-carrying protein in red blood cells. Fatigue, weakness, and irritability are the most common symptoms. Blood carries the nature of our own sufficiency; if our sense of who we are, nourished by the goodness of life, is lacking, chances are we won't have enough to share with the demands of another. Further, if one's Qi and Blood is squandered with busyness and taking care of others, this can only tax one's Blood further. Iron is a cool, sedating Yin aspect of Blood, which is required not only to supply the needed Blood to support pregnancy, but may also be required to cool excess Heat in the Blood. Iron equates with the Qi of action—the ability to do something with your life Blood.

Low levels are common during pregnancy, where there is a greater demand for blood and oxygenation. Low iron may result from low stomach acid or lack of vitamin C, and can cause pallor, fatigue, weakness, and dizziness, and can lead to depression, hypothyroid, and poor immune function, among other problems. Most women with iron deficiency anemia will already be taking an iron supplement, which can cause constipation. Iron-rich foods include shellfish, spinach, liver and organ meat, red meat, legumes, and pumpkin seeds. Iron deficiency is associated with Liver Blood and Qi vacuity. Vegetarians have a higher likelihood of developing iron deficiency anemia, as well as Qi and Blood deficiency. While the source must be addressed by modifying activity and continuing to build the Qi and Blood with formulae like Ba Zhen Tang (Eight Treasure Decoction) and Gui Pi Tang (Restoring the Spleen Decoction), when Liver Blood and Yin are deficient we can coax Wood with Lv 8 Ququan (Spring at the Bend) and Dang Gui Shao Yao San (Angelica and Peony Powder).

Rebellious Qi causing heartburn, morning sickness, or hyperemisis gravidarum

Constructing a fetus draws from the mother's Jing and Blood. The relative abundance of Jing and Blood required in the lower burner can easily cause a countercurrent between the Blood (below) and the Qi (above). This can create imbalance of the Stomach and Liver, and rebellious Qi of the Chong Mai. The Spleen, which must ascend to hold things in their proper place, may be weakened due to its job banking the embryo right now, and Wood/Earth imbalances may develop. The Stomach, which should be descending, might be irritated by certain foods that now cause Heat, irritating the stomach or esophageal lining. It's also important to recap how worrying weakens the Spleen; the Stomach could have difficulty digesting mom's new role as upcoming mother. There is such a thing as emotional indigestion.

Common symptoms include appetite fluctuations, heartburn, nausea, and degrees of vomiting, from mild to severe. It will be important to avoid energetically hot and spicy food and drinks, as well as Damp or Phlegm-producing rich or fatty foods. Too much sweet flavor can cause Dampness, which impairs Kidney and Spleen Yang.

Check for signs of Cold below and Heat above. Inspect the tongue for the location of Heat, and feel the pulses. If they are full, floating, and rapid, the imbalance is likely due to Stomach Fire. See if the right Guan pulse follows your finger down from the superficial to the moderate level. If not, you will need to clear Stomach Heat (St 44 Neiting (Inner Court), St 45 Lidui (Sick Mouth)) and descend rebellion (Ren 12 Zhongwan (Middle Epigastrium), Ren 13 Shangwan (Upper Epigastrium)). Wood may be insulting Earth, and Earth may also insult Wood. As Heat is siphoned away from the Stomach, it can go to the Liver and cause spotting. If the left Guan pulse is rapid and ascending, excessive Liver Yang must be settled (Lv 2 Xingjian (Moving Between)). Harmonize the Stomach and Large Intestine, (LI 10 Shousanli

(Arm Three Miles), St 36 Zusanli (Leg Three Miles)). Pc 6 Neiguan (Inner Pass) can harmonize the Stomach to alleviate nausea and vomiting. St 21 Liangmen (Beam Gate) can also be used to harmonize the middle; UB 20 Pishu (Spleen's Hollow), and UB 21 Weishu (Stomach's Hollow) should always be considered when the Spleen and Stomach are weak. Add St 40 Fenglong (Abundant Bulge) and spicy aromatic herbs that penetrate turbidity when Phlegm is present. Open the diaphragm with UB 17 Geshu (Diaphragm's Hollow). At this point in the pregnancy, most patients are still comfortable lying on their stomachs, but as pregnancy progresses, back points are accessed through side-lying treatments.

Also consider the three triangles or ten needle technique—the skeleton of the Li Dong Yuan's Earth School treatments when a weak Spleen is at the root of the nausea and vomiting. The following three triangles are needled in order, with the Conception Vessel points needled first, followed by distal points. Needles are removed in reverse order:

- Tonify Ren 12 Zhongwan (Middle Epigastrium), followed by St 36 Zusanli (Leg Three Miles) (stimulate until warmth is felt at Ren 12) to tonify the Spleen and Stomach function.
- Reduce Ren 13 Shangwan (Upper Epigastrium), followed by Pc 6 Neiguan (Inner Pass), evenly, to dredge Yin Fire.
- Tonify Ren 10 Xiawan (Lower Epigastrium) to harmonize the Stomach and regulate digestive Qi, then St 25 Tianshu (Heaven's Pivot).

The blueprint of the being's upcoming life is held by the Penetrating Meridian. The Gallbladder governs decisions, and if the child chooses not to accept this blueprint, the Penetrating Meridian may destabilize. Rebellious Qi of the Chong Mai interferes with the descent of Qi. Liver Qi stagnation may predominate this scenario, where Chong Mai rebels upward to invade the Stomach, preventing its Qi from descending. Sometimes the Heart Qi can't descend, which will be accompanied by vexation, and Blood may stagnate. Make sure you include Sp 4 Gongsun (Grandfather-Grandson) to fortify the Spleen, harmonize the middle, and regulate Chong Mai.

A great formula to harmonize the center is Su Ye Huang Lian Tang (Perilla and Coptis Decoction); to direct rebellious Qi downward—Ju Pi Zhu Ru Tang (Tangerine Peel and Bamboo Shavings Decoction). Xiao Chai Hu Tang (Minor Bupleurum Decoction) harmonizes Shao Yang; Ban Xia Xie Xin Tang (Pinellia

Decoction to Drain the Epigastrium) harmonizes the Stomach and Intestines when accumulation is present. Ban Xia Huo Po Tang (Pinellia and Magnolia Bark Decoction) when Phlegm is present, balance disharmony in the middle—warm Cold with Rou Gui (cinnamon bark) and add Huang Qin (skullcap root) to cool the Heat. When vomiting is severe, it will be difficult to ingest herbal decoctions, but sometimes fresh ginger (warming) or peppermint (cooling) tea can help settle rebellion. Strong smells can become especially problematic, exacerbating nausea and vomiting.

Hyperemesis gravidarum is a condition of extreme nausea and vomiting that can result in weight loss and electrolyte disturbances, hypotension, dehydration, and many other symptoms. Often the mother is extremely sensitive to smells and taste. Biomedicine has very little to offer to treat this condition, other than hospitalization to restore hydration and nutrients. While we still employ the appropriate measures listed above based upon the pattern, it is also important to remember that mom's Po might be reacting to baby's Po, or baby's Po may be having a reaction to the process of embodying. Here the Lung Qi doesn't descend, and may be pushing out the rejected Po. Lu 3 Tianfu (Heavenly Residence) calms the Po, Lu 7 Lieque (Broken Sequence) regulates the Conception Vessel, and UB 42 Pohu (Po Door) treats vomiting with agitation.

The Po is still capable of saying no to life anytime during the first trimester. Let's just say that All is One, and that Unity as Big Shen reigns supreme. It doesn't cleave itself into individual pieces and lose itself; every little cell within every little Pei and every mother participates fully in this grand process of embodiment. None is separate from any other. While we may not consciously be aware of it, if Shen as Po decides not to remain, Shen as the mother's body participates in this decision. The whole cosmos does. Remember, Metal asks only for more surrender. Perhaps our Po only meant to touch into this existence on its way to play as a meteor shower or a Tian Shi, an emissary from Heaven. The Gallbladder can help us penetrate between different realities. While our feet are walking in the physical world, we simultaneously live in the realm of spirit. One of the questions that supports the Gallbladder is to ask, *To which world do you belong?*

> Once Zhuang Zi dreamed he was a butterfly,
> a butterfly flitting and fluttering about, happy
> with himself and doing as he pleased.
> He didn't know that he was Zhuang Zi.

Suddenly he woke up and there he was, solid and unmistakable Zhuang Zi.
But he didn't know if he was Zhuang Zi who had dreamt he was a butterfly,
or a butterfly dreaming that he was Zhuang Zi.
Between Zhuang Zi and the butterfly there must be some distinction!
This is called the Transformation of Things.

—Zhuang Zi, Chapter 2

MOTHERS' GUIDELINES FOR THE SECOND MONTH
Nutrition

- Eat plenty of (cooked or sautéed) vegetables, especially soft, leafy greens.
- Ensure you are taking in adequate protein.
- Unsweetened, whole grain cereals can help sustain you.
- Eat green apples and lemon juice to help astringe and hold.
- Encourage your capacity to hold with thickening agents like cartilage, gelatin, and tendons.
- Stimulate bile with bitters—arugula, bitter melon, or chicory.
- If caffeine is a must, pu-erh tea in small doses relaxes the uterus, allowing more nourishment to penetrate.
- Avoid spicy, hot, or drying foods.
- Avoid fermented foods.

Lifestyle and exercise

- What arouses your senses in a positive way right now? Take time to rest and care for yourself, but also allow your own interests to be honored.
- Try refreshing new activities you haven't done before.
- Avoid being around strong scents, which can generate strong reactions.
- Honor some of your cravings and new eating habits, but try to continue to make healthy dietary choices.
- If you have any heartburn or nausea, try grounding practices; walk outside with your shoes off, if weather and location permit. Bring your awareness down to your feet. Massage your sole and instep.

- Set aside time daily to spend some time querying your body. How does it feel? Are there any sensations that want your attention? Your entire body and mind is housing your child, not just the womb.

Self-inquiry exercises

- The Gallbladder actualizes the Liver's dreams. What action do you need to take to realize yours?
- This month will benefit from decisiveness. Are there any areas in your life where you need to make a decision? What support do you need in order to make that decision now?
- Hesitancy and fear are considered "cold" emotions, which are not beneficial during this time. What fears hold you back from taking action?
- Emotions like anger, frustration, anxiety, and panic are "hot" emotions, which tend to upset the balance by over-stimulating. What is your greatest frustration or resentment right now? Can you journal about it, talk about it, or safely erupt a little bit to let it out?
- Emotions like guilt, shame, worry, and remorse are stagnant emotions that can be broken up by the Gallbladder. What are you willing to release right now?
- This is also a good time to strengthen weak personal boundaries. Learn to speak up for yourself if you need to. If your boundaries are overly rigid, practice softening and allowing more fluidity.
- Are there any conflicts between what you perceive internally and how your external life is expressed?
- Pay attention to your posture—how you sit, stand, and move in life. Psychological inadequacies and rigidities create postural changes. Notice any rigidity in your body, and see if you can mobilize it. Practice holding your body in different positions, and see how you feel.
- Your body must be able to uphold. What types of thoughts or feelings prevent you from holding yourself upright? Are you ready to release anything that drags you down? How can you become a little more flexible, a little lighter?
- As you move through your own issues, how are you helping to lighten the load for your baby?

CHAPTER 7

Pericardium: Lunar Month Three

Weeks 8–12

Days 57–84

> Yin and Yang are unified and refined,
> subtle, ethereal and immortal,
> self aware but not separate,
> inhabiting physical form but not attached to it.
> Guided by internal wisdom,
> the immortal embryo achieves wholeness.

The third phase of a being's life brings with it the rudimentary awareness that it is a distinct entity. This equates with early childhood, when the soul is still transparent and porous, prior to identifying with its conditioning. Since it isn't yet defined by *what* it is, it's still open to all possibilities. In one moment it could be a dragon; in another, a fairy. Before memory takes over and defines us by the past, we live in an imaginal realm where our orifices are still open. Toward the end of the third lunar month, from a primitive embryo, the pregnant uterus will bring forth a fetus. The Heart Master, Jingshen's internal connection with the Heart, is able to cleanse and purify the Shen. Now it can really become something.

Still in the realm of Po's influence over the first trimester, the Gallbladder pushes the embryo into another transition in the third month, governed by the

Pericardium, as Wood engenders Fire. As the mother moves into the second trimester, the coagulated Gao that has achieved some definition will now become a miniature person. At one level a "decision" was made in the second month; now it is accepted. As the physiologic foundational structure and rudimentary organs have been laid down, the soul accepts its upcoming life. With this "yes" to life, the basis of the fetal Po soul is established, and now it shall be purified so it will be ready to receive its lesson plan. This will allow the Shen to provide it with the three Hun, the basis of consciousness.

But first this Essence that inhabits the Pei has to be clarified. The embryo has its own Jing with certain genetic propensities, but it also has its own Heart-Mind, which endows it with the potential to live according to its precise divine plan. The Pericardium performs this purifying role so it may begin to be imprinted with humanness, a process called fetal education. It, like mitochondria, is provided by the mother.

Ancient Chinese societies were strictly matriarchal and loved their goddesses. Our beloved Kwan Yin was initially said to be androgynous, and could turn male or female at will. Nuwa, however, was the first mother goddess of creation. The male intelligentsia slandered her by suggesting she created humans by copulating with her brother Fuxi, but let's ignore that.

A bonafide wild woman herself, Nuwa sat at the river one day and began to shape humans out of the mud on the riverbank. And how she came to love her creations! Formed of the stuff of earth, they were also infused with her life-giving divinity. So more and more she made, swinging mud-dipped vines through the air that landed everywhere, as human droplets. Yet her creations didn't remain around forever; they perished after ten decades or so, and she'd have to start all over. So she divided them into Yin and Yang counterparts that would be drawn to one another so they could reproduce on their own. Now that the creation impulse was installed internally, would they lose themselves in the biological urge to procreate? Like any other mother, she had concerns. If she was no longer directly endowing her creations with awareness of their sanctitude at the onset, how would they come to know their wholeness? Her humans were still ensouled, but now it was their job to grow their souls into the light. To prevent their getting sidetracked, she constructed a temple in the center of their chests at Ren 17 Tanzhong (Center Temple), to remind them. This temple, which predated the Pericardium, contained the throne upon which the crowned empress sits.

Fetal education and gender

While biological gender is determined by penetration of the ovum by either an X or Y sperm, the expression of gender occurs during the third month. During the first month, the Qi and the Blood are at Ren 2 Qugu (Crooked Bone). During the second month it ascends to Ren 3 Zhongji (Central Pole), and during month three to Ren 4 Guanyuan (Origin Pass) and Ki 13 Qixue (Qi Hole, the doorway of the child). If you palpate Ki 13 Qixue bilaterally, according to Wang Su He, it may give you indications as to the child's gender. If it is more sensitive on the left, the form wants to become male, and if it's more sensitive on the right, female. The pulse is a relatively reliable gauge as well. While it is apparent soon after implantation, other energetic factors that will determine the distribution of Kidney Yin and Yang over the first two months might confuse, making the gender indications of the pulse less reliable. By the third month, however, some of the fluctuations will have settled down. When you compare the strength of the left and right Chi pulses, one side will usually feel stronger. If the left Chi pulse (Kidney Yin) is stronger, it indicates a boy is drawing from the Kidney Yang; if the right Chi pulse (Kidney Yang) is stronger, it indicates a girl is drawing from Kidney Yin stores.

Even minute amounts of estrogen at this time, found in much conventionally prepared food, water supplies, and skin products containing petroleum or plastic, may negatively impact a developing male fetus. Anti Müllerian hormone (AMH) appears in the developing male embryo, which prevents expression of the Müllerian (aka paramesonephric) ducts that become ovaries, fallopian tubes, vagina, and cervix. Instead, the Wolfian (aka mesonephric) ducts, which will become testes, prostate, penis, and the male apparatus, will be expressed. Testosterone is necessary to close the genital opening to push the penis and scrotum out. AMH will no longer be required during fetal development, but its presence will emerge again, when young women go into menarche. Once again it will hold back the expression of Yin. The greater the number of follicles that are developing, the higher the AMH to prevent multiple eggs from being released. We are not built for carrying litters.

The ancient Chinese believed that you could gender select during the third month based upon the mother's exposure to various influences. The more vigorous her activities, like archery and horseback riding, the more likely she was to have a boy. Doing dainty and pretty things, like playing with jewelry and putting pins in her hair, was more likely to produce a girl (or a very bored mother).

Today it is thought that the odds of producing a male or female child can be influenced around conception: intercourse closer to the release of the egg increases the likelihood of penetration by the more rapid Y chromosome carrying sperm, thereby producing a male child, whereas intercourse a few days prior to ovulation may predispose the more durable, long-lasting X sperm to produce a female child. But the mother's activities, her state of mind, and feelings all start to have an effect on the environment in which her child is developed. What was referred to as fetal education might be called epigenetic programming today.

Zong Qi and epigenetic programming

Our perception of our environment doesn't only control our hormones and behavior, but also the expression of certain genes. What we believe, consciously and unconsciously, filters certain frequencies that literally change our biology. The brain records what the senses take in, but the mind overrides the brain, excluding non-relevant data, and we perceive the world as we need it to be. The cellular membrane then picks up signals from the external environment and alters the cellular function to mimic our interpretation of our environment. What we perceive is then duplicated within; our genes, hormones, and neurochemicals are adjusted to fit the world we think we live in. Bruce Lipton (2016), has done extensive research, not only on the biology of belief, but also on how our beliefs and behaviors influence prenatal development.

Every expression in life is informed by the ancestral gathering Qi in the chest, Zong Qi. Our genes have coding and non-coding portions—that which is coded becomes information-transmitting Jing, while the non-coding portion becomes the Zong Qi, the epigenetic contributions that will determine which genes to turn on and off. Based on dietary and lifestyle factors, especially the mental and emotional influences of the mother, Zong Qi then can be seen as our ancestral and epigenetic influences. Most people understand that the food and drugs we consume impact the fetus, but few understand that just as important as the food we eat are the sights we see, the sounds we hear, the thoughts we think, and the feelings we feel. The fetus, of course, does not see what the eyes directly visualize, but its temperament will be influenced by the energies of interpretation that are carried in the Blood.

Whatever the woman experiences will produce a feeling state in her Heart. When she is around beautiful and harmonious environments, her Qi and Blood will tend to produce a more relaxed child. And if she is stressed, overworked, and argues with her partner, her stress hormones will educate her child to be more on edge. What she thinks about will filter into and influence the development of her child's mind. This doesn't mean, however, that she should become hyper-alert to every thought and feeling that crosses her mind, which will tend to produce more obsessive tendencies. It's okay to be sad and angry and worried at times. But the Shen that notices all these states likes to be calm, quiet, and non-agitated. And we always have access to these serene qualities, even when we are aware of other emotions. Fetal education begins with heart-based mindfulness, so you can create the patterning that will mold the child. If you want a happy child, expose yourself to happy scenes, that is, laugh a lot. If you want a generous child, be kind and giving. And if you want a competitive child, expose yourself to the inner chemicals induced by rowdy sports. The same is true of our own ever-developing consciousness. If we want kindness, we need to be kind. If we want peacefulness, we need to be that peace. Every postnatal expression will be informed by the same ancestral gathering Qi. Shen infuses itself into Jing, which lives itself out centrifugally as Qi, from this eternal moment on, defining each new direction life takes.

Wei Mai and happy babies

The Conception Vessel was established in the first month, the Governing Vessel in the second. During the third month the Penetrating Meridian harmonizes them, while the Belt Meridian embraces all three. This establishes the proper blueprint that the fetus will grow into during the second and third trimesters. Check for a "Chong Mai" pulse, which will be felt as a vibration at the moderate level across all three positions. This vibration could indicate the soul is not comfortable with its maternal environment; you may support the Chong Mai by needling Sp 4 Gongsun (Grandfather-Grandson) on the right, and Ki 19 Yindu (Yin's Metropolis) to help the Kidney to ascend to the Heart. If, however, the soul still doesn't accept its blueprint, the fetus may miscarry.

The third month also initiates the Yin and Yang Wei Mai (the Network Vessels), depicted as a silk net—an intricate matrix of cosmic nerve cells, where everything is interwoven between Heaven and Earth. This living web will become the time-keeper of life's rhythms, determining the cycles of development, maturation, and decline throughout life. The Network Vessels also represent how our blueprint, provided by Chong Mai, is shaped by life's unfolding. The Wei Mai are created in response to how we are socialized. When cultural conditioning goes against the dictates of our own blueprint, it leaves conflicts in the system and Wei Mai imbalances. Here we might have difficulty adapting to certain environments or be stuck in a certain unresolved time of the past. Wei Mai imbalances are like dropped stitches or knots in the fabric of our life story that weaken the bodily garment we wear through life. Yet Wei Mai treatments can pick up lost strands, and integrate tangled threads into a most interesting pattern. Baby's Wei Mai becomes more active, as its own Chong Mai blueprint starts to be activated by mom's conditioning.

Mythologically, the Wei Mai are represented by the ancient black tortoise Ao, who helped Pangu create the world, and Nuwa later restore the world. Ao's back holds up the world and her four feet are fastened between Heaven and Earth, symbolizing endurance, connectivity, and longevity, all with an easy-going nature as she patiently ambles across the universe. A metaphor of how everything is connected and nothing is isolated, Wei Mai, which knits it all together, can also be seen to represent how cellular signals are transmitted through receptors, and how rNA conveys messages to and from the cellular membrane and nucleic DNA. This brings us right back to how that which is not resolved impacts all other mind-body operations, and our beliefs impact the functioning of our genes.

Pc 6 Neiguan (Inner Pass) is the Luo point of the Pericardium, and the confluent point of the Yin Wei Mai; it is suggested to needle Pc 6 Neiguan and Ki 9 Zhubin (Guest House), the Xi-cleft point of Yin Wei Mai between trimesters (or any major life transition) to stabilize the curriculum. (Since we are in Pericardium's domain this month, wait until the end of the third month.) Together, these two points are referred to as the "happy baby" protocol, said to ensure a good-hearted child. At the beginning of the fourth month, and between the seventh and eighth, Ki 9 Zhubin harmonizes the host with the visitor, whether the visitor be a child, an exterior pathogenic factor (EPF), or some unresolved psychic haunting. These two points help transitions from one trimester to the next. Ki 9 Zhubin helps us to survey the cycles of major transformational periods of our life, bearing witness to our own inner process without judgment. Any unresolved past issues can be addressed here, harmonizing the Kidneys with the Heart. While Ki 9 Zhubin can clear the Heart and resolve emotional upset, it also prevents the transmission of maternal Blood toxins from the mother to the child. Uterine Heat that travels from the mother's Blood to the fetus may give rise to childhood diseases. Clearing fetal toxins can also be accomplished with Ki 16 Huangshu (Vitals Transporter). Further, moxabustion to Ren 5 Shimen (Stone Gate) is said to release "ghost children" from previous pregnancies that have died in utero, including when one child of a twin or triplet perishes, a condition called "vanishing twin syndrome," which, if not eliminated, can immunologically prevent future pregnancies.

Placenta and potential issues

While the corpus luteum has been busy manufacturing progesterone for the first 8 to 12 weeks of pregnancy, by the third month it hands the job over to the now functioning placenta, which becomes responsible for the production of the fetus's progesterone as well as other hormones, while also providing oxygen and nutrients and removing waste products through the umbilical cord. Once this newly functioning endocrine gland takes over, it's like the mother has her Spleen back: her energy levels usually increase and nausea and vomiting often diminish. A new Small Intestinal system of exchange is established where nutrition and information flow across a selectively permeable membrane with its own internal wisdom that determines what will be allowed to pass between mother and child. Through this intrauterine exchange, the fetus's cells migrate into the mother's Blood, a process called microchimerism, which imprints baby's live signature, *I was here*, on her tissues. Baby's cells circulate through mom's Heart and Blood, where she will continue to feel and know her offspring in her Pericardium.

Placenta previa occurs when the placenta overlays the cervix. As the uterus expands, the placenta and its vessels can cause significant bleeding during the latter half of pregnancy. While the risk factors include previous uterine surgeries leaving scar tissue, we view it as sunken Spleen Qi failing to hold the placenta in its proper place. The pulse should be assessed throughout pregnancy for proper Spleen ascension by checking to see if the right Guan pulse strengthens as your finger moves from the moderate to deep level. Address with Bu Zhong Yi Qi Tang (Tonify the Middle and Augment the Qi Decoction), UB 20 Pishu (Spleen's Hollow), Du 20 Baihui (Hundred Convergences), and St 36 Zusanli (Leg Three Miles).

Embryologic development

A cluster of cells in the fetal heart tube emits electrical signals within the pericardial cavity, which occupies the entire thorax. These heart cells initially congregate and start pulsing together. While the heart muscle won't be fully established until the second trimester, this single tube will begin to bend and spiral around until four chambers continue this synchronistic beat. Below the heart, there is an empty space, a real rarity in nature, that roots in the space between the Kidneys, and allows for the emergence of consciousness.

The heart develops along with the diaphragm, nervous system, and gut, foretelling the link between the Heart and Small Intestine, and the beating fetal heart initiates embryonic pluripotent stem cells that produce blood.

The Pericardium protects our innermost treasure, the Shen. It buffers traumas and extreme emotions that might upset the Heart. But a buildup of unexamined fears can barricade the Pericardium so much that it no longer feels. Overwhelming feelings and emotional passions, positive or negative, can cause upheaval in the system, potentially leading to Heat in the Blood, bleeding, or clots. The mother's unresolved traumas are passed on from her Pericardium right into her baby's Blood circulation during this time. This is why it is so important for her to reach into her deepest psyche, to recognize and resolve any protective mechanisms that she no longer needs.

The abdominal organs are formed, the bones begin to ossify, and the tongue appears to swallow. Circulation is beginning. The nervous system is becoming more complex as the neocortex is forming. The being's foundations have been laid; a certain identity is becoming. The fetal soul, which has also taken on Po influences from the cosmos and perhaps some contaminants from the mother, has to be purified so the Po can be established next month. As life is accepted, our little Pei moves into the fetal stage, becoming a Tai. Ready to receive its lesson plan, the Shen provides the three Hun during the third month. One Yin, one Yang, and one more human, these Three Hun will give rise to how the higher conscious mind functions in life. One carries the light that propels us toward our true heavenly home; one carries the light of our intellectual capacity; and one determines how we will be drawn like a moth to a flame toward certain life circumstances that will complete our curriculum. These three Hun spirits are always attuned to what we are doing in the container of time, swirling between past, present, and future, lifting us up like rising mist toward what we can become. While the three Hun spirits are imprinted during the third month, the seven Po spirits will enter next, which will provide exciting interaction for the Hun as they make their mark in full during the third trimester. But first, the fetus will spend the next few months being programmed by Shen.

Caring for the third month

This phase of development begins to establish consciousness in prenatal and self-consciousness in postnatal existence. The third phase of life is governed by Chong Mai, and the child knows itself as a distinct entity, separate from its parents, with its own life story, but probably not able to survive well on its own. It has to protect its own interests now. In utero, this corresponds to the stage at which the most rudimentary survival structures are intact, and while the embryo will be able to advance to the fetal stage, life outside the uterus still won't be possible. Unresolved issues from the third month will often show up in problems during the fourth month. This transitive property of karma will be the case throughout pregnancy.

Some of the concerns the mother might encounter this month have to do with how she is accepting this pregnancy and upcoming motherhood. As her child accepts life and moves into the next trimester, she has been making some lifestyle adjustments, too. Her body is changing. Her midsection is thickening and she has probably gained some weight. She may have to curtail some of her activities and may become more emotionally labile. The Pericardium directs movement, and emotions have directionality. The Pericardium has to adequately contain emotions or it can set up disturbances during the fourth month. We want to help curtail any excess rising, descending, or stagnation of the Qi mechanism by harmonizing the excess emotion and calming the Shen. While we will try to avoid Pericardium points (until we pull out Pc 6 Neiguan (Inner Pass) at the end of the month), we can utilize the second trajectory of the Chong Mai with the upper Kidney spirit points (Ki 22–27), or the outer Bladder line that addresses the spirit (UB 42 Pohu (Po Door), UB 44 Shentang (Hall of the Spirit), UB 47 Hunmen (Door of the Ethereal Soul), UB 49 Yishe (Abode of Thought), and UB 52 Zhishi (Will Chamber)). Any of the Heart points from Ht 3 Shaohai (Lesser Sea) to Ht 9 Shaochong (Lesser Rushing) can calm the spirit, as well as St 44 Neiting (Inner Court), when there is Stomach Heat.

Check the strength of the Spleen pulse, and as always, fortify if weak. Check for the strength of and communication between the Heart and Kidneys.

Treatment principles are to strengthen Kidney Yang, establish Heart and Kidney communication, and separate the pure from the turbid.

Harmonize the Yang Wei Mai to help Water contain Fire. Check for sensitivity beginning with UB 63 Jinmen (Golden Gate), traveling to GB 35 Yangliao (Yang Intersection), and then up to the Fire element at SI 10 Naoshu (Upper Arm Transporter) and SJ 15 Tianliao (Heavenly Crevice).

LI 11 Quchi (Crooked Pond) is recommended during the third month to clear Heat, cool the Blood, and regulate Qi and Blood.

You may add small amounts of Dan Shen (salvia) to cool the Pericardium if needed, and add Long Gu (dragon bone) and Fu Shen (poria root) to settle the Shen. E Jiao (ass-hide gelatin) may be employed if there is any spotting, but otherwise stay away from anything too sticky. While Dang Gui (angelica) can be used to tonify the Blood, avoid Shu Di Huang (rehmannia), which is a little too cloying at this time.

If the mother's Spleen is taxed, she has likely been fatigued and is sleeping more than normal. The increased circulation in the pelvis may give her hemorrhoids and cause her pelvis and legs to feel heavy. She may have a bearing-down sensation, especially if her Spleen Qi is unable to ascend, for which Bu Zhong Yi Qi Tang (Tonify the Middle and Augment the Qi Decoction) can be prescribed. She may experience bloating and constipation as well. Address the pattern and consider adding LI 11 Quchi (Crooked Pond), St 36 Zusanli (Leg Three Miles), UB 57 Chengshan (Mountain Support), and Du 20 Baihui (Hundred Convergences).

MOTHERS' GUIDELINES FOR THE THIRD MONTH
Nutrition

- This month it will be especially important to eat "clean," avoiding estrogenic-containing products found in many conventionally prepared non-organic food, water supplies, and skin products—petroleum products and plasticizers. Non-organic produce is often treated with xenoestrogens to keep pests from reproducing.
- Start to eat fewer, smaller meals throughout the day to decrease digestive upset and regulate blood sugar.
- Bitter greens like arugula, kale, and dandelion greens can help clear Heat and excess estrogenic build-up.

- Mushrooms help absorb toxins in the blood so they can be excreted.

Lifestyle

- Pay attention to what stressors remain in your life so you may reduce or eliminate them.
- If you watch television, stay away from scary, violent, or suspenseful shows.
- Do what makes you feel content and relaxed, but not lazy or lethargic.
- Practice daily gestures of self-nurturance—long, hot showers, watering the plants—whatever brings you peace and comfort.
- Reduce emotional extremes.
- Be as mindful as you can of your inner state. Bathe your baby in peaceful, loving feelings as much as you can.
- When you think about your child, what virtues do you sense he/she already possesses? Compassion, courage, trust?... What can you do to enhance these qualities in your own life?

Self-inquiry exercises

- Am I able to be soft and vulnerable?
- How have I protected my own heart from being hurt?
- What do I need in order to open my heart again?
- Have I accepted all aspects of my own life story?
- How do I or how can I trust in the inherent goodness of life?
- Do I trust myself, my partner, and my living situation?
- How do I experience joy and appreciation?
- How do I feel about this pregnancy?
- When I connect with my child, what types of qualities do I sense?
- How can I provide my child with the best internal environment to nourish these qualities?

CHAPTER 8

Second Trimester—
Shen (Fire)

THE ONE GIVES BIRTH TO THE TWO

We carry the secrets of nature within us. Albert Einstein said, *That which is impenetrable to us really exists.* And like a true Taoist at heart, continued to say that *behind the secrets of nature remains something subtle, intangible, and inexplicable*, a force which he venerated as his religion. Shen will infuse this subtle force into the fetus during the second trimester as a preprogrammed curriculum—not as in a book, but a song. Certain pitches of vibration will be transmitted through the Fu organs and stored in the Blood, establishing the themes that will give life meaning as it unfolds according to the time lines established during the third trimester. The Fire element dominated the third month and will sustain the transition to the fourth month and into the second trimester. We are one-third of the way through our journey, a good time to remind ourselves why we are here. Why are we inhabiting this life? Is it to find the Way and live the truth? After all, it's sometimes easier to submit to mediocrity or to try to make ourselves special rather than to live the authentic lives we were meant to live: deep, challenging, and immensely exciting.

Whether we are growing a child, treating pregnancy, or beginning life in utero, our souls are here to find the true Way, and will tend toward restlessness until they do. Joyful simplicity and cosmic harmony is the natural way. "True," authentic people, Zhen Ren, recognize that all is of the same origin. Perfectly reflecting the whole cosmos while remaining natural expressions of themselves, Zhen Ren were able to perceive the resonance underlying all things. Chapter

6 of the *Huai Nan Zi*, entitled "Surveying Obscurities," speaks of the concept of resonance, where the underlying subtle influence of all connected things is perceived by those who have attained the Way. All is in its proper place, guided by the movements of the sun and moon. There is no conflict.

Yet, when the Tao is lost, inherent virtues sour and we each go our own way. The pure Way becomes obstructed, setting off a series of events, seemingly unrelated but, in the web of life, nothing is. To get back to the Tao, we first have to stand back and survey where the kingdom went awry. This causality can be seen on a micro or macro scale. Think of the tyrant ruler, for example, who upsets the natural order of things, resulting in calamities like climate change and global havoc.

Earthly creatures were losing their sense of goodness and harmony. Their gratitude and reverence for life had previously nourished Pangu, who now was beginning to grow weary, trying to keep things in their proper place. As their spirits dimmed, so did Pangu's strength. One day the four pillars holding up the sky started to crumble, scorched by the blinding light of the burning sun. The earth caught fire, singeing its cracking surface, which let the floodwaters rise. Crafty vermin came out of hiding to prey on the people, who had lost the Tao and thus become weakened and sickly. Loss, it seemed, was imminent. The creator goddess Nuwa was summoned, for she still loved her creatures, although, as she feared, they had lost their way, they had forgotten they were the body of the Tao. Finding no answers in the clamor of the confusion, she looked past the stars to find her source, hidden in the darkness, and listened to the silence of the dark night sky, where all answers are given. She waited until she knew what had to be done. A difficult task was at hand. She called upon the ancestors to calm the winds down and then smelted five precious colored stones into molten azure rock to patch up the heavens. She took the legs from her beloved giant tortoise Ao to restore the four pillars, and sat upon its back, crying the oceans back into place. The world returned to peace.

Transitions challenge the natural order of what came before. As the embryo transitions into a fetus in the second semester, the mother undergoes her own transition as well. She looks pregnant now, and will be connecting to her child and herself in a different way. During this transition she can stand back to survey her own narrative, and change it if she wishes. When our own beliefs are challenged, it can create holes in the sky of our present mental understanding. The very ground we stand on can crumble until a higher order steps in to take the old one's place. But first we need to step into the unknown and dare to ask: what stories have we outgrown? What beliefs are we willing to relinquish in order to restore harmony within the queendom at hand? What challenges have transformed us into a more courageous version of ourselves? Are there any holes in our energy field that need to be patched up?

The first trimester explored how the Pei is fashioned within the realm of the seven Po deities who create any negativity for it to overcome; in this very necessary process, the mundane is made sacred. The innocent sage baby weaves precious golden coins, pressurized in the underground realm of our own fractured psyches, on a sacred golden thread to protect Tan Zhong, the temple in the center. We are ready to ascend higher. As the mother gives herself to the divine order, her offspring reap the evolutionary advantage. We give everything we have to purchase back our own souls. This is why we are here. We are in the realm of eight, abundance, but we don't stay here. Eight in the mist gives rise to a new power.

> When disturbed, I close the seven sensory portals and return to the peace and tranquility in the Heart where I give myself over to the Tao's whole making function. Here in the cave of renewal it is quiet and dark. Xuan, 玄 is the dark, obscure primordial beginning lying in wait to be brought into the light. Suspended in the mystery of inner darkness, the great ancestor and I are one. The moon rises within. The eight winds begin to stir; and blowing in from the eight directions, the eight immortals arrive to assist. I give birth to myself.

We have advanced from seven Po souls, Eight Extraordinary Vessels, and are now at nine, the realm of Spirit. While eight represents the extraordinary reservoirs, abundance, the eight directions of the I Ching, and the eight immortals that support the soul on its journey, nine represents longevity and sovereignty of the Heart. There are nine peaks on our journey that represent potential challenges created by the Xin (Heart-Mind). Our original nature, as seedlings of stars, must become wrapped in physical bodies like free birds enclosed in a cage, which will experience the release that comes when Shen is redeemed from Jing on our journey. We are here to live long enough to complete this task, whether it takes one or a hundred years.

It all begins in utero. Shen as Po has accepted life and the initial structures are complete, banked by Earth. The soul now graduates into the fetal form where Heaven begins programming the curriculum of its upcoming life. The unique markings of these principles will be stored in the Jing and Blood as certain strengths and weaknesses that will determine how the Source Qi will be distributed. The resultant tissue aberrations will become woven into the beautifully textured fabric of this individual life. As the mother's Shen is purified, baby benefits from her lessons, yet is relieved of her burdens.

Shen

> In peaceful calm, void and emptiness,
> the authentic Qi flows easily.
> Essences and Spirit are kept within.
> How could illness arise?
>
> —*Su Wen, Chapter 1*

Shen will imprint the child's curriculum during the second trimester, which will form its temperament. As such, it's important for the mother to focus on the qualities that make up a healthy Shen, so she becomes a clearer channel for the baby. As the soul makes its way, the *Ling Shu* stresses how important it is for all beings to attend to the spirit first. As it does so, the three qualities of Shen guide our health and wellbeing:

- Qi and Blood are harmonized to complete what we've set out to do in life.
- Communication between Ying and Wei Qi is unimpeded; there is no blockage between inner and outer worlds, no conflicts between who we authentically are and how we interact in the world.
- Curriculum has been completed at this point in one's journey, and the Zang Fu can express the highest virtues of each element.

If we are led too far astray by our animal instincts and any of these three qualities become deranged, we are prone to Shen disturbances. Transitions provide a potent time to survey and correct these disturbances. There are four cardinal signs of a disruption in spirit, when the mind function of Shen is disordered. It's important to note that the Shen themselves are not confused, except in relationship with the finite mind.

Shen disturbances show up as:

- Fatigue—or just being tired of life.
- Forgetfulness—life loses its meaning.
- Uncertainty—having no direction in life.
- Insomnia—a restless, preoccupied mind that can't relax.

These pitfalls can destabilize us as we aim to remain upright with our head over our heart over our heels, TaoTe 道德, as we walk through life. Te 德 is translated as power or "virtue." This virtue, however, is not referring to how your external behavior conforms to an ethical ideal; it is more intimate than that. Like the healing virtue of a plant, Te implies the inherent inner quality of a thing, or specifically, what it is that makes you *you*. The Te character combines a footstep, one's heart, and the radical for uprightness. When your movements reflect the integrity of your inner heart, you are following your true destiny, and your life will move with effortless cooperation with all you come into contact with.

We've inherited brains and muscles and organs, which are then culturally conditioned by our curriculum into neural pathways that become our life view. Some old pathways might be efficient, even when they no longer serve the highest good. Little Shen, held back by personal fears, tend to enjoy comfort and sameness. Yet the annoyance of our everyday habits can challenge us to break free of our previous casings, and, like a Phoenix rising out of the ashes, Big Shen emerges. We must constantly blaze new trails in order to develop feel good chemicals that stimulate our upward movement. Life is not meant to be all comfort and ease. Its goal is to return to the natural state, and often our states of dis-ease provide the fuel we need to rectify our unfinished business. When we default to our habitual neural grooves we become like Zhuang Zi's walking corpses. Life is an upward journey through which we must continually dive into deeper currents that propel us upward, like salmon into the rivers of life that birthed us, against the flow of entropy.

The spirits of Earth are Gui 鬼 (Po 魄 are white Earth spirits) and the spirits of Heaven are Shen. Together, the Gui Shen provide our life lessons. Shen 神 are extending influences from above, unseen powers that enliven us. Invisible, but very much alive, the Shen require stillness in order to be present. With a quiet Heart and mind, undisturbed by thoughts and passions, we are left with a simple sense of our own presence, our pure and uncluttered awareness. The more time we spend in internal quiet, the more the Shen come alive, and we experience their influence as a highly charged force with the power to rectify all. The art of the Heart is a Taoist practice to quiet the mind so the Shen can arise in the stillness of our own presence as gratitude for life as it is.

It is here that we are directed by the supreme heavenly deity Shang Di to follow our deepest, and most authentic, urgings as the Shen motivates the Qi and we radiate our highest vibrancy. As we come to recognize the subtle urgings of Qi, we begin to intuit the correct orientation of the natural movement of our lives through the four directions, the four seasons, and the eight winds. Like the eight directions of the I Ching, there are 64 possible combinations, like the 64 codons of DNA, the pattern that determines our body chemistry and how we see the world. The patterns are within, and the patterns are without—no difference. We learn to follow our true urgings, resisting the delusional nature of unrectified Po distortions and the subtlest secret of the Tao reveals itself in our very human nature. With our Heart-Mind set on the unitive principle, we let all things take their own course. We kindle the inner light in our own blessed land and there, hidden in the depths, Tao emerges, and our spiritual radiance shines through to guide us from within.

Curriculum

Picking up where we left off in the Po realm, in the 18th scroll of *Zhubing Yuan-hou Lun* (*Origin of the Etiology of Disease*), Chao Yuanfang spoke of nine types of worms associated with nine fundamental lessons, or Heart pains, themes that we are offered to transcend. These issues, often unconscious, when unresolved in life propel the motor that drives self-will. There are nine aspirations in life, which would ideally be balanced, but then there would be no movement. The eight winds are no longer at rest; as they rise, there is a new development. It may come as an outer pull or an inner push. Whatever the case may be, do not resist or these issues will recirculate and you'll have to come back and face them again. We each have a propensity to express a few or perhaps all of these urgings at different times, and some may devote almost their entire lives pursuing one particular area. Sometimes referred to as "Heart pains," they may cause psychological discomfort when we are in pursuit of or unable to achieve one. When these circumstances present themselves, we will be launched on our journey to summit one of the nine peaks (palaces):

Nine peaks or palaces

Wealth (sufficient resources)	Prosperity (reputation, honor)	Relationship
Health	Home (with oneself)	Children, creativity
Wisdom—inner knowing	Knowledge (vocational)	Global, world, travel

Don't assume that gestation automatically places one in the "Children, creativity" category. Some women have children to try to save their marriages (relationship), after overcoming life-threatening illnesses like cancer (health), or because they're afraid of not fitting in to society (prosperity). They can all overlap. When we enter a particular palace, peak, or Heart pain, we either highly value or resist associated issues, and may feel a great need to protect ourselves from related affairs. Qi depression may prevent us from taking the steps required to ascend the summit of our most troubling obstacles.

As you look at the chart, you may notice one particularly emotionally charged area where you spend more time or energy expressing or suppressing it than the others. This is your main peak. When you think about this present concern, is there a physical sensation associated with it? Does your heart rate speed up, blood pressure increase? Does it give you a feeling of warmth, a contraction in your gut, or tightness in the chest? Does your throat feel full like you need to swallow? Is there a sense of loss associated with it? Do you feel like you have to protect yourself or the issue? Then it may be a Heart pain, a peak that your destiny is urging your spirit to climb.

When these fundamental lessons emerge, there will often be a deep sensation that you are being threatened, that protection around this issue is required. This activates the Pericardium, whose job it is to protect that which the Heart holds precious. When you can open up to meet these issues head on, learn their lessons and transcend them, you have the possibility of reaching your destiny, intimately associated with your Heart's desires. Repressed Pericardium issues or long-standing Heart pains may need assistance through the unconditional love of the Heart and acceptance of the Lungs to open and release. You know what needs to be overcome. We all do.

When a Heart pain and its peak is overcome and its lesson learned, we have transcended one of the nine peaks in the crown, where Xi Wang Mu (Queen Mother of the West) resides. The highest peak for each of us is the first one—the challenge that we tend to return to the most. Through our own efforts, or those of other healers, we can't seem to get beyond these problematic juggernauts that bind us to our limited identities. If we are willing to surrender all that props up the false self, we are then picked up by the mythic bird that lifts us over Soul Vulture Mountain to enter the land of immortality, our true home. When we reach our own Kunlun mountain at the end of earthly life or the end of our egos, we can say, with assuredness, *I have completed my journey; my soul is my own.* The nine peaks are abandoned and we enter the purity of solitude. We are programmed for transcendence. We are meant to go farther than our forebears. We are meant to reach into uncharted territory, and to be heroines of our own life. And everything we need on our journey has been encoded in utero.

> You are the bows from which your children as living arrows are sent forth.
> The archer sees the mark upon the path of the infinite, and He bends
> you with His might that His arrows may go swift and far.
>
> —*Kahlil Gibran, "On Children"*

The container

The middle Dan Tien, which governs the second trimester, houses our Zong Qi where we are an extension of spirit through our biological and spiritual ancestry. Our temperament is encoded by pre- and postnatal relational dynamics that will establish our interactive life, our ability to set appropriate boundaries in relationship, and our emotional capacity to deal with others. Thus, most of our challenges in life stem from how we relate with others as we pursue what is most important to us. We are not meant to be perfect; we have all been marked by life. We have endured our share of challenges, and yet, we shine through with our own beautifully flawed markings. The pictogram for Li 理 depicts the principle of a thing, like markings in jade or rings on a tree, which provide its unique texture. Our highest guiding principle is to become more like ourselves, as the Tao intended.

The middle Dan Tien belongs to our humanity—the blending place of all—where we find that the shape of Tao is discovered in the shape of its manifestations, namely as a sense of *me*. My very being is seen as the shape of the Tao and it is expressed through awe and gratitude with an inflow and outpouring of the Heart. When I recognize the inherent virtue that Heaven in me is, the entirety of all of my life becomes a humble *thank you*—shifting the inner climate of my being into an offering of the fruits of the Heart—love, joy, and peace.

The *Ling Shu Jing* from about 940 CE shows this as the place where the fetus is suspended, hanging from the empty space below the Heart, where our true nature resides. In full receptivity it is ready for its curriculum to be inscribed by the master teacher, the Tao. Its only job is to receive. Its senses become attuned to the music of Heaven and an impression is made on its Heart. It must follow; there is no turning back.

MOTHERS' GUIDELINES ENTERING THE SECOND TRIMESTER
Lifestyle and exercises

- During the second trimester, energy should be returning, and most first trimester symptoms start to resolve, as the fetus's initial structures are complete.
- Your focus is now on maintaining a peaceful Heart, and participating in what type of temperament your child will have.
- Pay attention to foods and exercises that nourish and vitalize you. Do what brings you joy. Not excitement, but the quiet, peaceful joy that belongs to the Heart.
- Get out of your head, off your screens, and into your body. Immerse yourself in your life. Connect with your child.
- Spend time in nature, immersing yourself in creation. Reverently walk the earth, connect with its grounding nature, the womb of all that exists. Take in the abundant sights, smells, and sounds. Feel the sun, wind, and rain on your skin.
- Go out in the night sky, taking in the stars, the moon, and the blackness

that holds them all. Let the darkness speak to you of your origin. You are in the universe and the universe is in you.

- Attend to healthy relationships in your life; spend less time with people who aren't supportive. Are you able to receive help and support from others?
- Spend time in stillness every day, to allow any imbalances to harmonize within your heart. Darkness is not our enemy; it's our depths. As you spend time within, let your inner light shine through any darkness with the quality of vibrant aliveness that is your spirit.
- Notice what obstructs love and joy in your life. Through the Heart you can put old, worn-out things to rest, and through the Heart you can enliven what's been sleeping.
- If there are any past issues that cause you pain, see if you can rewrite the story you hold about it. Survey the image in your mind's eye with some distance. See all the players involved with impartiality. What support do you need to forgive and release?
- Be gentle with yourself; practice tenderness and self-care each day.
- Magnify the feeling qualities you want to impart to your child and circulate them from your heart to your uterus. Feel your child receiving these qualities.

Daily review to clear the palace
Each day provides an opportunity to clear out and release any unfinished business. Before bed, review your day, scanning from dawn to dusk, remembering any thoughts and feelings that stand out. Was there any sense of fear, anger, worry, anxiety, or regret? Is there anything you felt you should have done but didn't, or anything you did but wish you hadn't? Any troubling feeling or judgment that remains is an invitation to revisit the event and recreate the memory without trying to fix the feeling or change the situation. Just allow it to be. On deeper reflection, could you have actually done anything different? Is your perception of the event "true," or did it occur exactly as it must? Which elements belong to your life story and which have been inherited? Can you glean any wisdom out of this situation so you can let it go and move on? As this becomes a practice, your Heart-Mind becomes cleansed of its troubles so you can sleep in peace and awaken fresh and new each morning.

Meditation for the Shen

Close your eyes, and bring your awareness to your Heart space. Spend some time noticing your breath moving in and out as it facilitates the circulation of Blood throughout your body. Relax deeper and deeper. Tune into the feel of your own beating Heart. While you may not hear it with your ears, feel it with your inner listening. This is the first sound your child will ever know; it is the echo of the first sound you ever heard, tucked safely in the womb of your own mother, listening to her heartbeat. It was the first sound she ever heard from her mother, and her mother, and all of the mothers back to the very first mother.

Feel your Heart open—first to yourself, and then to your child. Now, with an even deeper listening from the ears of your soul, can you hear the faint echo of your ancestors who hold you suspended in this plane? Open the ancestral door of your Heart to connect with loved ones no longer walking the Earth who can help nurture you, your child, and your ancestral line. Tune into a deeper community of voices who are here to support you. Feel their breath in your breath, their blood coursing through your arteries. You are alive with generations. Take in their love for you and your child. Occupy the place of infinity, where you hold the portal open that they may help carry the energy that is to come. Feel its vibration, and if you are so inclined, give it voice. Hum, speak, or sing to your child with these vibrations to remind it how much it is loved and cared for by all of creation. And feel your child taking it all in.

CHAPTER 9

Triple Energizer: Lunar Month Four

Weeks 12–16

Days 85–112

The Ming dynasty physician Zhang Jie Bin, author of the Leijing (類經) and Jingyue quanshu (景岳全書) calls Mingmen the Fu of Water, the ocean of Jing Qi and the passageway of life and death from which the San Jiao distributes the Yin and Yang of Water and Fire. During the very dynamic fourth phase of life, Yin and Yang divide, and the process of separation is always challenging. Part of the being becomes more alienated from itself, but because it never fully divides, it paradoxically becomes *more* of itself. This is an important part of any metamorphosis; a teenager has to stretch out and find out what they're not, to discover who they are. Likewise, as the fetus (or a human brain) develops more complexity, it seems to be distinguishing itself from the void and everything else. Yet it's just a change in focus, as nothing can separate from the Tao. During the active fourth lunar month of pregnancy, the Triple Energizer, through its internal connection with the Fu, will also be busy composing the Blood vessels.

In our process so far, the combined Jing have embraced, calling in the Po. Wood has initiated the decision to proceed, which the Pericardium has accepted. We have now officially graduated to a fetus 胎, whose pictogram is composed of the flesh radical 月 and its support system 台. The simple form, which looks like a house, is actually composed of a mouth exhaling a breath, which means to be able to make oneself known, to have an "I" to speak. As the pregnancy enters into the fourth month, we have some major work to accomplish; we have the rudimentary structure laid down, but now there is an "I" to enflesh, a life plan to allocate, and vasculature to distribute.

Moving Qi of the Kidneys and the distribution of Yuan Qi

The left Kidney encapsulates our foundational Water constitution, and the right Kidney expresses Ming Men, the Fire of activity that brings vitality into substance.

Between the two, at Du 4 Mingmen (Gate of Destiny), Ministerial Fire contacts essential Water—right where the threads from Heaven are attached—and generates a swirling energetic current, the cosmic residence of Shen and Jing, and the doorway of our individual destiny. And with a force that spins galaxies, essential Water meets Ministerial Fire, and essential Qi is produced. The *Nan Jing* refers to the Source theory where Yuan (Source) Qi is disseminated by the Triple Energizer, which belongs to the Fire element, and distributes each element to the corresponding Bladder Shu points.

This month Source Qi, the precursor of every other vital process in the body, is pumped up the spine to begin distribution into the twelve meridians. Not belonging to the five elemental phases, the basic and "highly respectable" Qi of the Triple Energizer provides the power that propels the movement of life. Now the Fire official accepts the first of the five agents, Water, with all of its unique characteristics, and allocates its Essence to the Kidneys, reflected laterally at UB 23 Shenshu (Kidney Transporter). Associated with Water Jing during the fourth month, the fetus is endowed with the compressive energy of fear, which precedes new movement.

The Triple Energizer, it is said, has no form—only function, and its initial function is to allocate the unified left and right Kidneys' essential Qi up the ladder of the spine, to the back Shu points in a certain unique way, never to be repeated in another human being, ever. The *Nei Jing Tu* (*Chart of the Inner Warp*) depicts this process as four swirling Tai Chi symbols in front of the passage of the Milky Way in the low back, where we could say essential Yin and Yang are subdivided into young and old aspects creating the four symbolic representations that make up the eight trigrams and 64 hexagrams of the I Ching that parallel the 64 DNA codons, the very warp of life. It's beginning to become an "I."

If some of the activity described above seems like a repeat of conception energetics, it is. That which was established during the first month now spirals back to extend the same note, only an octave higher, during the fourth month. This energetic process repeats itself throughout life. The Tao gives birth to consciousness/Shen; consciousness then gives birth to self-consciousness/me, and then self-consciousness finds its way back to universal consciousness. While the child won't be conscious of itself as a distinct "I" for another year-and-a-half or so, subconscious tendencies are being epigenetically programmed through the Zong Qi, which will have the propensity to explode in about two cycles of seven.

Remember your own stage of adolescence where you were becoming an "I" who was trying to make herself known—to others and to herself? For the mother, this is the flavor of the month. This is an optimum time to reclaim any neglected or confused aspects of your teenage self. The baby, on the other hand, will need its own encouragement. The mother can convey that she sees and recognizes her baby, an important dynamic to begin practicing now, even if it is just through emitting a felt sense to the baby. *I recognize you.*

The Mawangdui transcript says that in the fourth month the prosperity blossoms to make the eye and ear communicate and the meridians and connection circulate. The Heel/Motility Vessels (Qiao Mai) link up the Kidney energies from the bottom of the foot with the brightness that shines out of our eyes (where we step out with an independence of spirit to become who we were created to be) with the power of Shao Yang to which the Triple Energizer belongs.

Fetal maturation

The Triple Energizer (San Jiao) elaborates and extends, reaching and forming connections. Chapter 62 of the *Nan Jing* says, *The San Jiao has its source in the original qi or the Ming Men, and acts as the intermediary between destiny and all the functions of the body emerging at the Yuan Source points.* The initial process is established now, while throughout postnatal life, the Yang Triple Energizer will help guide this ongoing process by working hand in hand with the Yin Pericardium to regulate our expansive drive to share our destiny and connect with others, while reinforcing our boundaries so we don't become overly vulnerable or lost to others.

Formation of the six bowels (Fu), conduits of human connection between Heaven and Earth, is emphasized during the fourth month. The Celestial Qi descends, to be received by the bowels, which transmit downward from above. Like Heaven rains down from above, the six bowels transform, drain, and do not store. Unlike the solid Zang organs, the role of the Fu organs is to fill and empty. Yet, in utero, not yet charged with filling, their only roll is to receive. The Triple Energizer receives directly from the Gate of Destiny, so the spiritual force can be distributed up the Bladder's inner line, making up the innate constitution.

Fetal neurologic activity is now also heightened as the brain is learning hundreds of billions of neural connections to synchronize vital functions. Skeletal structures strengthen, teeth appear, and the ears are capable of picking up sound. As the internal organs develop further, the peritoneum begins to wrap around them and extend to the extremities as the original formation of the twelve-channel system, all governed by the Triple Energizer. Through this, the solid Zang organs extend to their corresponding external orifice. Blood vessels proliferate. Our fetus has gone through the reptilian and mammalian evolutionary stages and now has a distinct human form.

Five agents of Jing enter—Water Jing is accepted

The basic heavenly Qi, which provides the implicate order for the unfolding of life, will be distributed unevenly into the pathways that comprise the emerging nervous system and initiating the five elemental agents. Like a live Tree of Life, the developing Yin organs will receive these via the control cycle as Water/wisdom, Fire/trust, Metal/order, Wood/kindness, and Earth/integrity. Each enter in varying degrees to establish the individual constitution, beginning in month four with the essence of Water and ending in month nine with the essence of Stone, which heralds the completion of fetal life. Since Water is the first element that the Triple Energizer will distribute, and the first to be accepted, the Kidneys tend to become weaker during the fourth month. While the Triple Energizer commences the distribution of the constitution, during the next five months the rest of the agents of Jing will enter one by one. How the mother cultivates these virtues during each corresponding month maximizes the fetus's ability to absorb each one respectively. Thus, this month she should expose herself to wise and philosophical works.

Luo vessels develop

With the Triple Energizer nourishing it, the fetus develops a more complex nervous system—the makeup of which is somewhat like the image of a miniature Banyan tree, where stems and branches grow upright, while aerial roots shoot downward to provide more sustenance. In the same way roots absorb water and minerals, which the tree transforms into sap, Essence is now becoming the Blood of the developing fetus. Essentially reversing the process that was established in the first month where Liver Blood supported the production of Kidney Jing, now Jing will be used to create Blood. During the fourth month the vascular Luo vessels begin to develop. The fetus creates these Blood tributaries as needed to handle the overflow that will emerge as its essential Qi unfolds into life challenges that will affect the Blood level. Because Blood will be distributing those star seeds of the Shen flowing through our vessels to enliven every cell, it is wise to keep our Blood as charged as possible with this life-giving force. Luo vessels are therefore established first, creating the framework to handle any toxic or psychic overburdening of our precious Blood resources.

During the fourth month, the mother's unfinished business can easily become her baby's as the fetus absorbs her Fire toxins. Pernicious familial and psychological issues in her blood can be transmitted into the baby's Jing. As the fetus is creating Luo vessels, fetal toxins can show up on the surface as birthmarks or moles. The mother may also develop skin discolorations resulting from changing hormone metabolism. A dark line, referred to as linea negra, may appear on the Conception Vessel line below the umbilicus from Ren 2–8, and she may develop an increase in freckles around SI 18 Quanliao (Cheek Bone Crevice), both of which indicate Blood stasis. The Liver may become taxed trying to keep up with the changing estrogen metabolism. If Blood-deficient, the mother's body may be trying to hold on to the now stagnant Blood. During this time her child is developing Luos, she may concurrently develop varicose veins.

Shen provides Jing with the seven Po, which carry rudimentary mood states that might appear at any moment. These moods will develop into more complex emotional movements with the establishment of Blood, which begins to contain the seven emotions. Emotions, like the Blood, can be nourishing. Love and gratitude fill the heart, but terror and aggression can injure the Blood. Fear at this time may be especially damaging to the fetus. While it is virtually useless to tell someone not to have the fear that they're having, since Earth controls Water, we can use reflective thought to keep fear in check as we talk someone through their fears. The sage is watchful and attentive to her interior life. This interiorization, proper to the darkness of winter, implies looking inwardly. When she can see past the fear, the virtue of Water, wisdom, is born.

Caring for the fourth month

The Book of Elixir describes how "the hen can hatch her eggs because her heart is always listening". This implies how the energy of the Heart penetrates into the depths to quicken the life within, whether it is an immortal embryo or a fetus.

The energy of the Heart penetrates into the depths to quicken the life within.

The soul's impressionable consciousness is becoming more susceptible to epigenetic influence through the mother's heart. If she is worried and fearful, her baby will be more likely to turn on the genes that encode for those traits. Fear is especially damaging this month. Needling SI 19 Tinggong (Palace of Hearing) can turn listening inward to concentrate the spirit and infiltrate the palace of potential. While San Jiao disseminated the Source Qi up the inner Bladder line, the outer line provides the associated spirit. To strengthen the Water element and baby's Zhi, consider gently stimulating UB 22 Sanjiaoshu (Triple Burner's Hollow), UB 23 Shenshu (Kidney Transporter), and UB 52 Zhishi (Will Chamber) to maximize this reception.

San Jiao takes constitutional beliefs held in the dense Jing and transforms them to a gaseous state where they are raised to the heart so the wisdom of Shen can challenge those that aren't true. The Triple Energizer can be used to relinquish belief systems that have been engrained in the Jing, especially those that effect self-worth.

The Triple Energizer also regulates our external connection to the world. Like a well-functioning thermostat, the Triple Energizer makes sure there is a corresponding change inside for every change outside and vice versa. So the fourth month, when San Jiao dominates, should be a time of minimum fluctuations lest Cold and Heat impact the developing circulatory system, causing inconsistencies in how the fetus is patterned. The mother should remain calm and undisturbed. Severe agitation can harass the child's Heart, potentially showing up postnatally as Attention Deficit Disorder, Obsessive Compulsive Disorder, or Autism Spectrum Disorder.

Treatment principles include strengthening the Kidneys and their ability to support the Heart. Movement from the Kidneys to the Heart is represented by Rou

Gui (cinnamon bark) and Gui Zhi (cinnamon twig). Small amounts at this time may be called for, and cinnamon makes a nice tea, especially in colder months.

Ren Shen (ginseng) and Dang Gui (angelica) will be useful to help tonify Qi and Blood. Add Da Zao (Chinese date) if there is loss of appetite. Ju Hua (chrysanthemum) helps clear heat in the San Jiao and Ban Xia (pinellia) can help clear fullness in the chest. Gui Zhi (cinnamon twig) can help promote sweating. Jin Gui Shen Qi Wan (Kidney Qi Pill from the Golden Cabinet) may be appropriate to tonify the Kidneys. Ki 9 Zhubin (Guest House) will continue to protect the child from any toxins the mother may transmit, while LI 11 Quchi (Crooked Pond) will help cool the Blood and regulate the bowels. If the mother becomes tired after meals, St 36 Zusanli (Leg Three Miles) can tonify Qi and address any digestive issues and rebellious Qi.

Low back pain and body pain are not uncommon during this time for which you can tonify the Kidneys and the Source Qi. Utilize Ki 3 Taixi (Supreme Stream), UB 63 Jinmen (Golden Gate) to clear the channel, UB 22 Sanjiaoshu (Triple Burner's Hollow), and any sensitive Bladder Shu points. As the pregnancy progresses, these symptoms may be exacerbated for other reasons. If you don't have a pregnancy adaptable treatment table, make sure you have appropriate bolsters; as her belly grows, mom will be more comfortable in a side-lying position during treatments.

The Triple Energizer brings Fire and Water together. As Jing is being converted into Blood, Heat and Cold intermingle, which can create a temperature inversion. It may bewilder you to find Heat settling in the lower regions and Cold above. GERD (gastroesophogea reflux disease) and esophageal reflux, often associated with Heat, may now be accompanied by a contracting chest tightness; this month it will more likely be due to Cold rising. Here we will have to warm the chest with Moxa to move the excess. Heat can also be displaced downward, producing signs usually associated with Yang vacuity, like frequent urination, abdominal pain, and distention. Since Heat is attempting to displace the Cold this month, we will need to clear excess Heat before tonifying Yang. Urgent sensations around the navel that rush into the chest (Running Piglet Qi) causing anxiety and panic can indicate that there might be vascular stress in the child. Address this by opening the Chong Mai with Sp 4 Gongsun (Grandfather-Grandson) and pairing it with Pc 6 Neiguan (Inner Pass).

The mother may also experience chest distress, stiff neck, and atrophy of the elbows around the He Sea points, a metaphor for stiffness in the bowels. It is extremely important to disinhibit and regulate the bowels, as any constipation will cause her to retain and transmit toxins to the fetus, tucked right in her underbelly, receiving both messages from Heaven and waste products from Earth. The mother should therefore consume more roughage, and we can prescribe Yin-supporting moist laxatives like Zeng Ye Tang (Increase the Fluids Decoction) to encourage the bowels to move. Use St 36 Zusanli (Leg Three Miles), St 37 Shangjuxu (Upper Great Hollow), St 39 Xiajuxu (Lower Great Hollow), and Ll 11 Quchi (Crooked Pond) to address the Stomach, Small and Large Intestine, and invigorate the Blood with UB 17 Geshu (Diaphragm's Hollow) or Sp 10 Xuehai (Sea of Blood).

Because of all of the activity going on this month, and the potential to release toxins into the circulation, it isn't unusual for the mother to experience flu-like symptoms in conjunction with a detoxification healing crisis. It may appear as a Wind-Cold type presentation; if Yang isn't strong enough to release the exterior to push the toxins out, chills will be stronger than fever. Tonify Yang and help release exterior with Rou Gui (cinnamon bark) and Gui Zhi (cinnamon twig). Strengthen the Kidneys with tonics like Jin Gui Shen Qi Wan (Kidney Qi Pill from the Golden Cabinet) or Liu Wei Di Huang Wan (Six Ingredient Pill with Rehmannia), or nourish the Jing with seeds (Fu Pen Zi (Chinese raspberry), Gou Qi Zi (Chinese wolfberry), Tu Si Zi (cuscuta), Wu Wei Zi (schisandra berry), Che Qian Zi (plantago seeds)) to help move these poisons out. The mother is also advised to eat scaly fish like trout and salmon to help absorb the toxins that the fetus would otherwise inherit. Wild goose is supposed to initiate a healing crisis to get rid of any Fire toxins. Clear and harmonize with points like UB 11 Dazhu (Great Shuttle), Lv 14 Qimen (Cycle Gate), Sp 10 Xuehai (Sea of Blood), and UB 17 Geshu (Diaphragm's Hollow). Ki 9 Zhubin (Guest House) prevents the transmission of maternal toxins to the child, and Pc 3 Quze (Marsh at the Bend) can clear Heat from all three levels. Heat and toxins may produce autoimmune reactions and the mother may be found to have elevated antibodies. Clear heat with Ll 11 (Crooked Pond), Sp 10 Xuehai (Sea of Blood), and Fire points from affected channels: Ki 2 Rangu (Blazing Valley), Lv 2 Xingjian (Moving Between), Sp 2 Dadu (Great Metropolis), and Lu 10 Yuji (Fish Border).

Look for Luo vessels and varicosities. They may be on the Bladder and Kidney channels around the ankle or along the organs that have already been activated. Look especially around Lv 5 Ligou (Woodworm Canal), GB 37 Guangming (Bright Light), Pc 6 Neiguan (Inner Pass), and SJ 5 Waiguan (Outer Pass), and bleed them.

Moxa SJ 5 Waiguan to release Fire toxins. As always, simultaneously tonify and move Blood.

If sleep patterns, postural issues or poor self-esteem arise, harmonize with the Qiao Mai, including UB 62 Shenmai (Extending Vessel), Ki 6 Zhaohai (Shining Sea), and UB 1 Jingming (Bright Eyes).

Encourage light exercise and perform a squeeze-and-release type massage in the mother's arms and legs to stimulate the vascular system.

MOTHERS' GUIDELINES FOR THE FOURTH MONTH
Nutrition

- Non-glutinous rice and grains like oats and barley should be eaten now.
- It is also advised to avoid acidic juices, soda, and carbonated beverages.
- Increase your intake of fiber and prebiotics like chicory root, dandelion greens, Jerusalem artichokes, onions, garlic, leeks, bananas, apples, asparagus, and flaxseeds, to name a few.
- While you shouldn't have to supplement with probiotics if you are eating right, probiotic foods like unpasteurized sauerkraut, miso soup, and unsweetened yogurt or kefir will help your bowels remain healthy.
- Include scaly fish like trout and salmon to help any toxins absorbed in your system to be released.
- Mushrooms also absorb toxins.

Lifestyle and exercises

- The focus this month is on (you guessed it) more balance and harmonization.
- Avoid extreme fluctuations—hot, cold, stress, loud noises, arguments, and activities or events that you find frightening. Anything that overly agitates you will also harass the heart of your developing child.
- Get adequate light exercise, but avoid getting overly stimulated, which can agitate your child.
- Spend time in solitude and get plenty of rest. There is a lot going on under the surface this month.

- Consciously conserve your Qi. Get to know and honor the energy you inhabit.
- Change your position a lot. Stand a while, sit a while, walk a while, lie down a while. We want to avoid excess movement, but this will prevent stagnation.
- Get compression-type massages to encourage blood flow.
- Pay attention to your posture—to how rooted your heels are and how high you are carrying your head. Does your stature convey the respect of your own life? With your feet anchored on the ground, feel your instep lift. Straighten your spine and lift the top of your crown to the sky. If your mood is low or you are feeling more wide than upright, lift your gaze and see if it changes your outlook. Slight adjustments can make big changes to the inner environment.
- Listen to music that stirs your soul. Sing the song of yourself to your own inner ears, and let it penetrate into your child's ears.
- Reading thought-provoking books—pondering the grandeur and mystery of life, and having philosophical discussions can bathe your body mind and new creations with wisdom, the virtue that is most active this month.

Self-inquiry exercises

- Notice what causes any fear that holds you back from living fully.
- When you feel fear, don't fight it. Just notice what it does to your system and do what you can to return to a feeling of safety.
- If lack of self-esteem or poor self-worth is part of your history, how can you treat yourself with dignity, and act with estimable behavior?
- How able are you to keep your Qi and Blood inside to nourish yourself and your child? Start to notice what and who depletes your energy.
- Chart your life priorities. List the five most important things in your life. Place yourself in the middle and draw five circles. Place each of these items in a circle, making the size of the circle proportionate to how important it is to you. Draw those things that are most present in your life in close proximity to you at the center, and those things that are more distant further away.

- Journal about your experience charting your life's priorities. Without judgment, notice what your priorities are.
- Does your energy expenditure line up with your priorities?
- Spend time in your body. See if you can feel a sensation like the warm glow of a pilot light in your low back. This area is referred to as your Gate of Destiny. Allow it to open up and communicate with the area around your heart. Then allow the energetic current to open between the low back and uterus, and between your heart and womb. Circulate this energy like a triangle between these three energy centers.
- Wisdom is an attribute of the soul, rather than acquired knowledge, and it requires an open mind. See if you can glean any insights from the being inside you about the realm of the unborn. Are you both being held and supported by the love of the universe in the same way?

Spleen: Lunar Month Five

Weeks 16–20

Days 113–140

St. Symeon, instructs us to use the intellect to search inside ourselves "so as to find the place of the heart, where all the powers of the soul reside". The fifth phase of postnatal life begins the process of solidifying the adult identity. The being is, it knows that it is, it has tested its boundaries, and now it can say: *this is what I am.* In our sojourn through Earth School, the soul is inextricably drawn to certain people along the way. Magnetic charges draw us to situations (nine peaks) that are part of our curriculum. Yet oftentimes we make our homes in these peaks, defining ourselves by them rather than learning from them and moving on. As we progress through the fifth phase of life as an adult, we trade our expansive infinite potential for smaller and more defined limitations: *This is me; this is not me.* The adult tends to identify with its roles to tell it who it is. If attention is only given to the character's performance as mother, partner, friend, or professional, it creates a smoke screen over the awareness of its innate beingness. While it once knew its true name, if it's defined only by its place in the world, it will feel bereft, like something's missing. But before we become too set in our ways, we have the opportunity to ask, *What have we learned thus far on our journey? How have the roles we have played defined us? Which don't fit anymore? Which roles have to be defended? Which can be relinquished?* And finally, *what is your significance to yourself if you don't refer to any of the roles you play?*

The fifth phase of life correlates well with the fifth lunar month of pregnancy, where the process of solidification begins. Leg Tai Yin, which controls the four seasons, completes the four limbs and composes the Qi, which thus begins to be utilized in more predictable patterns. In accordance with the control cycle, the essence of Fire begins to be accepted this month.

We are halfway through our ten-month journey, and the uterine fundus reaches Ren 8 Shenque (Spirit Palace Gateway), the midpoint on the way to the summit at Ren 14 Jueque (Great Palace Gateway). The Essence that created Blood's Luo vessels last month now turns toward Qi production. Heaven will begin to chisel tissue chambers for new energy flow this month, which the Spleen will compose. The Spleen produces the Blood and the Blood from the newly developed Heart contains Shen. While Blood and Water Jing unfold through the Triple Energizer, the essence of Fire is accepted this month to produce the Qi that will accomplish the work established by the essence of Water in month four. The Po provide our challenges; the Blood holds them; and Qi imparts the ability to handle those life experiences. After producing the Qi, the Sovereign Fire of the Heart distributes it to each organ's command. It is Fire that ignites our passion, that sings of a quiet joy, and grants us the warm glow of peace.

Essential Qi gives rise to the matrix of the primary channels. Qi is the mother of Blood and the Spleen produces postnatal Qi. The Triple Energizer etched the initial foundation for the primary channels last month; now the skeleton of the primary channels will begin construction, starting with the Zang in month five and moving to the Fu in month six, defining how this new being will take on some of the challenges in its foundation that previous generations have left behind. These are not to be rejected; most of us are already plagued with a sense of not belonging. It all belongs; previous misunderstandings are meant to be incorporated into this new structure, and the Spleen manages integration by weaving it all together.

> So vast! No one knows where they ultimately end.
> So broad! No one knows where they finally stop.
>
> —*Huai Nan Zi, Chapter 7.1*

We each harbor a blending of ancestral lines that reach all the way back to the origin. We inherit our unique structure, talents, and shiploads of whatever it took to survive. Unresolved trauma along the way may arrive in this body-mind as a sense of *something's wrong*. We are still consolidating energies this month, so it's a ripe time to synthesize anything that feels cut off from our center of being so we don't unwittingly pass it on to our offspring. Attentive awareness is the key here, not analysis. Like Rumi's poem, "The Guest House," we *welcome and entertain them all! Even if they're a crowd of sorrows who violently sweep your house empty of its furniture, still, treat each guest honorably. He may be clearing you out for some new delight. The dark thought, the shame, the malice, meet them at the door laughing, and invite them in. Be grateful for whoever comes, because each has been sent as a guide from beyond.*

In this month of integration, we may become better versions of our past selves by taking in all that we've been given—whether or not we embrace it, we can accept who we are. When we cease to be divided within and become unified, integrity results. Sometimes the strongest alchemy is simply allowing our little irritants that aggravate the system, like sand in an oyster shell, to just be present and acknowledged and ultimately transformed into pearls of great value.

During the fifth month, Zong Qi influences the baby's developing temperament largely through the most recent ancestral conditioning—the mother's physical and mental health, which, thankfully, is still able to be directed. After birth the process of influencing Jing/constitution and curriculum will be modulated by familial and societal conditioning, but for now, it percolates in the mother's Qi and Blood.

Ancestral survival instincts are genetically transmitted, conveying the information that helped our ancestral line adapt to the changes in nature they encountered. They survived with whatever they were given, and so do we. We aren't our own faults. We can't know where "we" begin and end, because we don't begin or end. We are Shen involved in an exchange of Qi further back than we could ever know. While some inherited instinctual patterns may no longer serve us, we can accept them, honor them, thank them, and only then can we change them. If we resist them we can be assured they will be transmitted onward; nothing resolves through suppression. This is the month where we can either courageously bring them to light within our selves, or pass them on.

You, my child, do not belong to me
anymore than I do.
We owe our being in part to the spirits that paved our way.
Every strand of 'me'
I've simply picked up along the way—

birthmarks of ancient wounds.
My grandmother's shame wraps my heart
along with her exquisite care.
A hunter's fierceness rises up my spine.
The envy in my ribcage I don't recall putting there
but it's mine to wear just the same, mine to overcome.
My child, we have work to do,
lifetimes of incompleteness to attend to.
I take off my outgrown costume; as my self unravels
I wrap myself in the garment of the Tao.
Stitched of birch bark, forgotten dreams and twinkling stars
it fits us perfectly.
We belong.

The mother's Qi movements affect her offspring, especially now, when the four limbs are being completed. As the Qi begins to manifest in the fetus, it begins to move and quicken. Mom may feel the first kick. While we looked at posture and external energy distribution last month, now we can evaluate and challenge internal energy leaks by evaluating the movement of Qi through our present life movements. Is the Qi distributed equally throughout the head, heart, gut, and limbs? Does more go to the surface than the core? Are forward-initiated movements (Tai Yang) synchronized with the ability to stop the momentum of previous movements (Yang Ming)? Where do we need to shift and pivot (Shao Yang)? What beliefs and behavioral patterns deplete or stagnate the flow of energy? Any imbalances can obstruct the free flow of Qi and Blood, potentially manifesting in pain conditions.

Fetal maturation

The fetus accepts the essence of Fire during the fifth month. *At five months it is complete... The five flesh are already created, then the nine orifices occur. The Spleen occurs at the nose, the Liver at the eyes, the Kidneys at the ears, the Lungs at the [other orifices].*

The five sensory organs are completed, and the baby begins to recognize sounds now. It can discern and bond with the mother's voice. The half-in-the-cosmos, half-embodied being can communicate with the mother through her dreams; it may even tell the mother its name and share its logos, its identity.

The five Zang organs are completely formed, although their functioning will have to mature. As such, the fetus can differentiate the five tastes. Mom's Spleen now gives the fetus the ability to distribute its essence to the five Zang. Any cravings she has may reveal any strained or deficient organs.

The Kidneys begin to consolidate, and the bones and tendons solidify. With the formation of the primary channels, the fetal limbs stretch and extend. It has lots of space in which to move around in order to strengthen new neural and skeletal connections. As its movements are felt, mom feels baby as a definable being now, who is beginning to move in particular ways at particular times. This is an expression of the newly establishing temperament, which will be reinforced through continued conditioning, environmental factors, and life experiences.

Caring for the fifth month

Blood, which has been fortified in previous months, is the mother of Qi, and the Qi of the Heart should be quite exuberant this month. It will be important to support Yang without adding excess. As the essence of Fire is received, Yang may become over-exuberant, manifesting in rapid pulses, excessive sweating, and body odor. Heat may rise to produce upper body symptoms again. Because of the excess Fire energy, avoid overstimulation with strong acupuncture and moxibustion; gently massage or lightly needle acupoints. If too much Yang is generated, the Qi that produces the primary meridians can scatter away; yet you can temper the Fire by strengthening Water. If Fire remains uncontrolled, it may result in Heart defects, including emotional instability; other structural or genetic deformities may begin to be exposed at this time as well.

Harmonize the center and stabilize the Zang organs this month. The fetus is consolidating, so mom's Qi needs to be protected. Check the status of the pulses for Qi distribution, and reinforce any weakness by Moxaing the source point. Strengthen the Spleen to help keep things together. The Spleen controls the Yi, which provides concentration. Heat distracts concentration, which may make mom become confused or prone to short-term memory loss. She may displace her car keys, pocketbook, forget appointments. Stabilize the Heart, which may be confused and disoriented.

Tend to the Spleen–Heart relationship. If the Spleen doesn't have the power to produce Blood's red substance by ascending to the Heart, she may be slightly anemic—this could mean Qi or Blood deficiency. Support the quality of Qi; the energy around her should be clear and clean. Mom needs to absorb more Qi (while not overheating) and keep from drying out. She is advised to go outside in the morning to absorb sunlight, but not when it gets hot out. Decoctions are going to be favored over pills and herbal concentrates. Sticky herbs like Long Yan Rou (longan) and decoctions like Gui Pi Tang (Restoring the Spleen Decoction) may be helpful. Harmonize the five flavors. Use ascending herbs for a weak Spleen (Sheng Jiang (ginger)), descending herbs like Hou Po (magnolia bark), and Zhi Shi (immature bitter orange) if the Stomach is weak. Harmonize with Gan Cao (licorice). Warm the center without causing too much Heat with herbs like Tu Si Zi (cuscuta). Sun Si Miao recommended An Zhong Tong (Cardamom and Fennel Formula) to calm the middle and augment the Qi. Restless limbs can manifest due to Qi/Blood's inability to anchor and keep up with the growth requirements. Supplement with Ba Zhen Tang (Eight Treasure Decoction) or Si Wu Tang (Four Substance Decoction). If restless limbs are due to Heat, use Huang Qin (skullcap root). E Jiao Tang (Ass-Hide Gelatin Decoction) is still best to address any bleeding, and add Xuan Fu Hua (inula flower) to help anchor the Yang to the Kidneys and stabilize the Fire.

The mother may continue to experience digestive symptoms, heaviness in the legs, and hemorrhoids. Last month's pain conditions were most likely related to strained Kidney energies; various pain conditions can manifest this month as a reflection of how her Qi is able to distribute to the fetus and herself. As the developing infant's energy is extending to the limbs, hers may be compromised. For achey and restless limbs due to unrooted Qi, regulate with Ki 5 Shuiquan (Water Spring), and consider UB 63 Jinmen (Golden Gate), UB 20 Pishu (Spleen's Hollow), and UB 49 Yishe (Abode of Thought). SI 11 Tianzong (Heavenly Gathering) addresses shoulder, chest, and breast pain, and can also help call to the ancestors should mom need support with familial issues.

If there are signs of a restless pregnancy, Ki 9 Zhubin (Guest House) in combination with GB 13 Benshen (Root Spirit) can be used to calm the fetus.

Gestational diabetes

Gestational diabetes usually manifests after 24 weeks gestation, but when we understand its mechanism, we may be able to prevent it. The development of Xiao Ke (wasting and thirsting disorder) can be due to malfunction in the San Jiao mechanism. Insulin is the storage hormone that represents Spleen's transformation (Qi) and transportation (Yang). During pregnancy the body isn't in sugar storage mode, but its metabolism shifts dramatically to keep up with the increased energy demands. When the placenta is fully functional, it releases human placental growth hormone to block insulin's Yang action on the cells, thereby increasing blood glucose levels in order to supply the higher demands for Qi and Blood. This interferes with the insulin's Spleen Yang-like action of driving glucose into the cells (insulin resistance), which can cause blood sugar levels to rise too much. Glucose is a sweet, Yin substance that provides the Yang energy that all cells need. Yet too much sugar taxes the Spleen Yang's ability to drive it into the cell to be utilized, quickly turning to Dampness, stagnating Yang movement, and causing Heat. Together, increased insulin and glucose creates a damp, sticky environment with unstable Yang, often on a background of underlying Qi or Yin deficiency as well as depressed Liver Qi.

Our first line of defense always begins with dietary modification, consuming foods with low glycemic index. Assess the status of Qi and Yin, and make sure Heat isn't building up. Ensure adequate Qi and Blood circulation without upsetting the delicate balance of Yang. Tonify underlying Qi or Yin deficiency (rehmannia formulas like Liu Wei Di Huang Wan (Six Ingredient Pill with Rehmannia)), clear Heat, and if draining Dampness, simultaneously incorporate herbs with an upward effect like Sheng Ma (cimicifuga), Jie Geng (platycodon) and Huang Qi (astragalus). Heat due to Liver depression can respond to Dan Zhi Xiao Yao San (Free and Easy Wanderer) with additions. In more severe cases, Xue Fu Zhu Yu Wan (Drive out Stasis in the Mansion of Blood Decoction) can be used to harmonize the Liver and Spleen while gently moving the Blood to guide out stagnant Qi. In addition to treating the pattern of imbalance (staying away from Spleen points this month if you can), use UB 17.5 to regulate blood sugar located ½ Cun below UB 17 Geshu (Diaphragm's Hollow). If the mother starts to get light-headed, dizzy, fatigued, is unusually thirsty, or urinating frequently, address the pattern and recommend supplementation with a regimen of chlorophyll evenly spaced throughout the day, and add chromium picolinate, N-acetylcysteine, bitter melon, and fenugreek as needed, to keep blood sugar levels stable.

MOTHERS' GUIDELINES FOR THE FIFTH MONTH
Nutrition

- Continue eating whole grain cereals that you may supplement with brewers yeast (high in selenium, B vitamins, and chromium).
- Keep eating vegetables, fruits, seaweed, and high-quality protein sources.
- Include asparagus, high in chromium, which can help stave off blood sugar fluctuations next month.
- Make sure your diet contains adequate dairy or calcium-rich foods.
- Warm soups will be helpful, but not too hot—try tendon soup, which many pho restaurants carry, to help strengthen your tendons and ligaments.
- It is recommended to eat moist, sticky foods like sticky rice to keep from drying out from the heat this month.
- Try to avoid drying foods like dried fruits, which the body has to hydrate.
- Stay away from deep-fried, smoked foods, beef jerky, or dehydrated vegetables.
- Make sure you expand your diet to include all five flavors—salty, sour, bitter, sweet, and acrid. It will be best to combine them—sweet and sour, etc.
- Cravings and food aversions can let your acupuncturist know of any strained organs, and it might help to share a food journal with them.
- Caffeine will be too agitating for the baby's needs this month. While you might feel fine, it is not good for the baby's energy.

Lifestyle and exercises

- Sleep in late and get plenty of rest.
- Absorb more Qi by getting out into the sunlight, and bathing yourself in warm water, but don't use hot tubs, saunas, or direct heat application.
- Avoid spending time with people you don't know or whose energies you have to accommodate.

- If you wake up hot, do gentle Qi Gong exercises to vent the excess Yang energy.
- Throughout the day, try a full body shake for a couple of minutes to release tension.
- Shift your routine daily movements to prevent fixated patterns. Walk side to side or backwards. Reach into the cupboards with your non-dominant hand. Squat to reach lower shelves. Move your body the way your baby wants to move.
- You may find yourself sweating and smelling a bit more ripe. Bathe and change clothes often.
- You have been practicing communicating with your baby. This month allow your baby to communicate with you through your dreams. Keep a dream journal, noting any feelings or images that appear significant.
- If you haven't "picked out" a name, see if your baby communicates its name to you.

Self-inquiry exercises

- What aspects of yourself do you trust or distrust?
- How can you maximize trust in your inherent goodness?
- What roles in your life no longer serve you?
- Which are you ready to relinquish?
- Do any obsessive thoughts recycle through your mind?
- What type of experiences do they create for you?
- Can you identify any underlying fear behind them?
- Which beliefs do you feel you have to defend? What does the defensiveness do to your system?
- Is there any part of your physical, mental, or emotional makeup that feels like it doesn't belong—that perhaps you've neglected, rejected, or suppressed? Can you share this with your practitioner or someone you trust, and ask for help accepting it?
- Do you recognize any physical, mental, or emotional patterns that originate in your ancestral lines? Which do you embrace and which do you have difficulty embracing?
- Is there any part of your ancestry that has been rejected, or feels like it

doesn't belong? What can you do to honor it and integrate it into your life today? What aspects do you fear might come forth in your child?

- What ancestral issues need forgiveness?
- Do you feel resonance with any of your ancestors? How could you open up to guidance from them?
- Body scan: Sit or lie down. Pause, breathe, and turn your attention inward. Notice where most of your Qi is located—in your head, heart, belly, feet, hands? Allow the energy to equilibrate simply by being present to it.

CHAPTER 11

Stomach: Lunar Month Six

Weeks 20–24

Days 141–168

> Your true face
> is made of the eternal dance of dark and light.
> It hides as a wave and it emerges as a particle.
> Xuan Nu (the dark lady) made it in the image of her dazzling darkness.
> You'll see mine when you know your own.

The sixth phase of life brings us into the peak of adulthood, where our conditioning settles in to become a well-defined identity. The way we see ourselves determines the view we have of others and how we respond to the world. During early life our true nature is ever-present, but not consciously known. After being battered around a bit trying to be who we are and who we aren't, to act correctly according to societal norms, all while saving face, we end up perceiving the world as we see ourselves and listening mostly to the sounds of our own thoughts. In the sixth phase of life, when our identities are relatively concretized, our views also tend to become more hardened. Just as sediment accumulates in the bowels impairing their digestive function, the window into our true nature can crust over and we forget the heavenly tone imparted this month in utero.

Zhuang Zi says the perfect mind is like a mirror. It grasps nothing, regrets nothing; it stores but does not keep. When you have lost the firmament of your own divine home, return to the bowel's evacuation function and empty the mind of self. Plunge your awareness into the gut and listen past your thoughts.

Listen to the emptiness. Even if it is a faint echo in a forgotten cave somewhere within, try to recall the music of the spheres that resounds deep within you. Breathe deeply into the gut to restore the original timbre of your own unique and guttural Om. Begin humming, drumming, or whistling along, even if you're out of tune; it gets easier with practice. Rehearse daily or as often as you can. There is no better use of your time.

Correspondingly, in the sixth lunar month of pregnancy, Leg Yang Ming energy influences the mouth and eyes of the fetus and composes the muscles of the leg. The Spleen's function of *banking the fetus* wrapped up the previous five months of consolidation. While these two months of Earth continue to solidify, in the sixth month the Stomach will take over with its bright Yang to get the fetus moving. Let's look at the dynamics Yang Ming brings.

Recall that the bowels are empty conduits that receive from Heaven and pass on to Earth. While the Stomach gives rise to physical hunger, the soul craves something more difficult to satiate. It is said that during the second trimester, Heaven blows six pitches of vibration through each of the newly developing Fu organs. The Stomach is the grand Fu organ, on which Shang Di plays a unique song of the soul like a celestial calliope, reminding each of their original nature. These tubes are conduits of emptiness, nutrition, and the soul's call back to itself, an ancient anthem in which we all long to participate. Like the gurgling of a hungry gut, an inner melody intones somewhere deep within, waiting for us to pick up its pitch and become chambers of its resonance.

Where the Conception Vessel accepts the initial responsibility to sustain life, the worth and dignity with which we accept this human existence is the Stomach's domain, exemplified by St 9 Renying (Person's Welcome)—how we receive and welcome our own humanity. The Stomach meridian runs from the eye to the mouth and around the jaw before plunging into the gut, representing the rudimentary reception between our environment and our sensory apparatus. It is the pathway through which information enters the body, before we assign meaning to it. The Stomach is basic for survival; the whole of our flesh wraps around this tube that breaks things down for initial processing, out of which our physical body, especially the musculature, will be fashioned, since the Stomach is in charge of digesting protein.

The Stomach's rotting and ripening process conveys the idea of breaking things down so they can become something else. The way we absorb information and synthesize experiences prior to personally ascribing any emotional significance is the Stomach's psychological equivalent. The Spleen, on the other hand, provides meaning. In the same way Gu Qi becomes Blood, experiences, fully assimilated, become our life story, a summary of ideas upon which our beliefs and view of life are based. Too much or the wrong type of food, information, or stress simply can't be absorbed. When input exceeds the Stomach's capacity to process, digestive disorders, abdominal fullness, and cluttered thoughts are likely to ensue. We could say the Stomach receives each event purely without context—it notices, *there are clouds.* Then the more complex Spleen steps in to define what it means for the individual, interpreting based upon beliefs and associations. *Cloudy days are depressing because I have seasonal affective disorder.* Therefore during this month, seek simplicity. Eat smaller meals. Move a little more. Limit sensory exposure.

As the musculature develops, the Qi has to maintain the tonicity of the spine and musculature. The fetus's movements are more forceful and the mother feels them more. The sixth month is when the Sinew meridians nourish muscle function and set the stage for the development of the divergent channels. The fetus is learning to move around and perceive the world via the mother's vision. With a lot more eye activity going on, she may develop vision problems this month, especially if her Liver is strained. Metal Jing is now accepted. Mom's sense of order and correctness might be challenged this month as Metal holds our judgment. She may become more critical and opinionated this month—and if it's strongly expressed, this may cause her remorse.

As movements become more complex, we need to know how to correct our course should we lose our bearings. As the mother rectifies her Qi, so does her baby. The Stomach is the origin of Wei Qi, and also provides the Jin fluid necessary to support Wei Qi's functions. The fetus now receives Metal Jing, whose essential Qi is Wei Qi—Wei to engender the development of the skin, the sinews, and the space between the skin and sinews known as the Cou Li space, governed by the Lungs. Cou 腠 is depicted with the organ radical next to the representation for trinity and humanity, over Heaven. And Li 理 is the principle or underlying texture of a thing. The *Jin Gui Yao Lue* (*Essential Prescriptions from the Golden Cabinet*) says that the Cou is the space where Yuan (original) and Zhen (true) Qi converge in the Triple Energizer, and that Li is the pattern of the Zang Fu. So our basic source and our most refined genuineness meet in this triple layer of defensive Qi, along with the dynamic means by which we must protect our innate vulnerability Qi surfaces from external influences. Li also means to put in order, to set things right, or to rectify, another function of Metal. And Metal deals with our insecurities, the things we feel we need to protect. It goes against our very survival instincts to show our weakness, so we may take actions that protect our psychological survival in order to save face. Unfortunately, these behaviors often go against our conscience, and the Qi and Blood suffer. Unresolved issues can stagnate in the Cou Li space, which, protective by nature, can be difficult to access.

Later in life our most challenging issues might leave us with the residue of remorse or guilt—the unresolved feeling that we should have handled ourselves or the situation another way. While we couldn't and we didn't, it still sticks in our craw. And if we don't do some psychic scouring, our feeling of doing wrong, being wrong, gets passed on. The same goes for our parents, grandparents, and the entire ancestral line. While nobody could have done anything differently, each of us has the opportunity to resolve how these challenges show up in our lives here and now.

Guilt, a sense of wrongdoing governed by the Lung, and shame, a deeper sense of being wrong belonging to the Stomach, can only corrode our vibratory patterns, and both of these organs' energies must be optimal this month. Some of us harbor such a sense of remorse that we feel we don't deserve to let go of the offense and move on.

Forgiveness, a Metal virtue, is its remedy. When we accept our past human failings (part of how the Stomach accepts our humanity), we release the Qi that was bound up in the past (Metal) and free it up to move differently and create new patterns. While Metal creates order, Qi rectification is a function that includes the Spleen, which fortunately became dominant last month. The Stomach moves interiorly, the Lungs move exteriorly, and the Spleen occupies the center where rectification takes place. We are put back in proper order, and regain ourselves.

We began with Water Jing in the fourth month. Since Water controls Fire, the Fire Jing was active during the fifth month. Fire controls Metal, and Metal Jing enters this month. Thus, if the fetus is most active this month, it will likely be born with a Metal constitution. This is the time to establish Metal virtues like discernment, judgment, and a critical appreciation of the arts. Metal provides order, but when our conditioned ways of viewing life become overly solidified, our body and mind tend toward rigidity. As Metal Jing is accepted, the white lightning of Po proffers the celestial gift of our deepest challenges. The seven aspects of the psyche can potentially torment and corrode Metal, but if we know we are here to learn from them, they can also provide the alchemical fuel by which our darkest issues are transfigured into the pure white light of spirit. Courage is a primary virtue to carry us though our Earth School curriculum to assist our souls in reaching toward the heavenly light of spirit.

The Spleen banks the Blood, providing our worldview, and how we will act it out; the Stomach digests and assimilates; and Metal defines. The order established by Heaven will solidify the fetus into its proper place this month as it becomes more distinctly itself. Its face, as well as its Metal tendencies, are being etched from the inside by the Master Carpenter's tools.

As the Cou Li space strengthens, the fetus' features start to fill in. Cou refers to the lines on the skin, like wrinkles and fingerprints, and Metal imparts definition as well as the face the baby will show the world, which will determine at least partially how others will respond to it. Toward the end of the month, the baby will be able to make and change facial expressions, which will become more complex next month.

The fetal form has achieved completion, and the baby could potentially be viable if born now. While the baby has been swallowing amniotic fluid and practicing sucking and chewing movements for weeks, this month peristalsis begins, as the Stomach prepares to descend its Qi. The Stomach also provides the fluid substrate for muscles and sinews to develop, making movement intensify. The baby will be tumbling and turning in response to inner and outer cues.

The baby can now hear sounds that originate outside the body. Prenatal ultrasound waves vibrate at frequencies higher than the naked human ear can detect; however, through the uterine tissue and amniotic fluid, the baby can hear its hum. If close to the baby's ear, it can be more like a shout, as loud as a blender, causing agitation and distress. Considered standard diagnostic tools, ultrasounds provide no direct benefit to the baby or mother's health, and it is the mother's prerogative to make decisions for her baby.

Caring for the sixth month

We are past the midway point of pregnancy. The mother may be bearing not only excess weight, but also the responsibility of motherhood, which might manifest as back pain. Her skin and surface areas may begin to be reactive and she may feel vulnerable, insecure, and emotionally labile. If you've ever been six months pregnant, weepy, and insecure, you don't necessarily want to talk about it, and nor do you appreciate platitudes about looking at the sunny side of life. Nothing in particular may be wrong. She may just need to cry. And sometimes practitioners just need to allow it, providing the quiet embrace of spirit that allows water to rise to the eyes and wash the upper orifices. Then the emotional release can be tempered, so she doesn't strain the Qi.

The sinews, governed by Wood, may hold tension of her pregnancy and other unresolved matters, which the Liver can rectify by releasing stagnant Blood. The Spleen, dominant last month, also assists with Qi rectification. Sp 4 Gongsun (Grandfather-Grandson) rectifies our relationships with our ancestors; Sp 8 Diji (Earth Pivot) ascends the red substance to the Heart to rectify the Blood, which holds our emotions; Sp 12 Chongmen (Rushing Gate) rectifies imbalances when our internal blueprint conflicts with family dynamics; Sp 17 Shidou (Food Hole) rectifies our relationship with food. And when we feel stuck, Sp 18 Tianxi (Heavenly Stream) rectifies our place under Heaven.

Rituals can strengthen Metal's ability to serve as divining rods to connect us to our inner holy places. Alchemists like Ge Hong performed ritualistic acupuncture to serve this sacred function. For example, connecting Ki 12–15 bilaterally and linking them up with Ren 8 Shenque (Spirit Palace Gateway) forms a vortex of energy around Ki 13 Qixue (Qi Hole, the doorway of the child), and invites excess emotional energies and attachments to be cleansed and rebirthed. Because it is now filled with child, however, you could instead invite excess emotional energies into the chest where the Heart and Lungs can release them. We can then anoint these points (Ki 12–15 and Ren 8 Shenque) with essential oils like rose, lavender, or frankincense to enhance the healing effect. Forming a figure "8" between Lu 1 Zhongfu (Central Palace) and Lv 14 Qimen (Cycle Gate) (alpha and omega) resets any disrupted day/night rhythms. Further, we can return to our Nine Flower treatment to address any diaphragmatic and abdominal fullness (Ren 14 Juque (Great Palace Gateway), St 19 Burong (Not Contained), Ki 19 Yindu (Yin's Metropolis), Ki 21 Youmen (Hidden Gate), and Ki 23 Shenfeng (Spirit Seal)).

From this month on, we want to facilitate movement (rather than consolidate), and Qi tonics may help resolve lassitude; if prescribing tonics like Ren Shen (ginseng), also add Huang Qin (skullcap root) to clear any resultant Heat. Mom's legs may be feeling heavy. If Spleen ascension is weak and she is experiencing any bearing-down sensations, small amounts of Huang Qi (astragalus) or Sheng Ma (cimicifuga) can help ascend the Qi along with St 36 Zusanli (Leg Three Miles) and Du 20 Baihui (Hundred Convergences). Huo Xiang Zheng Qi San (Agastache Powder to rectify the Qi) and Mu Xiang (aucklandia) help harmonize the middle and rectify the Qi.

You may find floating pulses, as the essential Qi is going out to create the sinews. If they are weak and floating, however, especially in the right Cun position, there probably wasn't adequate Qi support last month to efficiently move out to the Wei Qi level this month. Thus, the mother might develop gestational tendinitis like carpal tunnel or De Quervain's tenosynovitis. In addition to local points around the wrist, use GB 34 Yanglingquan (Yang Mound Spring), the influential point of the sinews to nourish the tendons and indirect Moxa to SI 18 Quanliao (Cheek Bone Crevice) and Ren 3 Zhongji (Central Pole).

As Metal Qi is allocated to the fetus, the mother becomes more susceptible to exogenous pathogenic factors, so she will need to be covered up, warm, and adequately hydrated. Because the sinews are developing, there will be more movement going on now, yet too much movement can deplete the Yin. Dehydrated muscles spasm and tremble. Nourish Stomach Yin to support Lung Yin, which supports the Cou Li. Mai Men Dong (ophiopogon) is the main herb to support Lung Yin; Ge Gen (pueraria) can release the muscles and generate body fluids while Jie Geng (platycodon) can guide it to the upper body. Relax the muscles of the spine and shoulders to help fluid circulate. Lymphatic massages and passive foot-pumping motions can encourage fluid movement, which will become more important as pregnancy progresses. Lu 7 Lieque (Broken Sequence) should be used to strengthen the Lungs and reinforce the Conception Vessel.

Abdominal discomfort

The mother's center of gravity is changing; her breasts and belly grow, adding frontal weight to which the spine curves in response; abdominal muscles stretch; ligaments and joints are loosening and may become more easily strained; there may be more pressures on the nerves; and tissues may become engorged.

As Qi and Blood are diverted to support the fetus, Qi may stagnate, making mom feel crampy and irritable. Choose from Lv 3 Taichong (Great Surge), Lv 14 Qimen (Cycle Gate), SJ 6 Zhigou (Branching Ditch), Pc 6 Neiguan (Inner Pass), UB 13 Feishu (Lung's Hollow), UB 18 Ganshu (Liver Shu), and UB 23 Shenshu (Kidney Transporter), and consider prescribing Xiao Yao San (Rambling Powder). Blood deficiency may cause the uterine vessel to become empty, which may also make her feel unrooted and restless. Here Lv 8 Ququan (Spring at the Bend), St 36 Zusanli (Leg Three Miles), UB 17 Geshu (Diaphragm's Hollow), UB 18 Ganshu (Liver Shu), UB 20 Pishu (Spleen's Hollow), and UB 23 Shenshu (Kidney Transporter) may be appropriate. Herbal formulations may include Dang Gui Shao Yao San (Angelica and Peony Powder), Ba Zhen Tang (Eight Treasure Decoction), and Jiao Ai Tang (Ass-Hide Gelatin and Mugwort Decoction). This pattern can be complicated with Blood stasis, which will intensify the pain. Add Sp 10 Xuehai (Sea of Blood) to the Blood-deficient points and add gentle Blood movers to the above formulas. Mom may also experience empty Cold with an underlying Yang deficiency. She will, of course, feel cold and may also lack any vitality. Moxa Ki 5 Shuiquan (Water Spring), Ren 12 Zhongwan (Middle Epigastrium), St 36 Zusanli (Leg Three Miles), and UB 23 Shenshu (Kidney Transporter), and prescribe Jiao Ai Tang. And as always, address the spirit, perhaps with Yintang, Shenmen, and Shishencong.

Urinary issues

Urinary leakage becomes more common as the pregnancy progresses and puts more pressure on the bladder. Kidney and Spleen Qi need to be strong enough to overcome this tendency.

With fluid being diverted to the sinews, the body may attempt to hold on to its reserves of Qi, Blood, and body fluids. While the etiology is empty in origin, as the mother tries to retain fluids, they tend toward turbidity and stagnation, leading to urinary retention or urinary tract infections. Her lower abdomen may be uncomfortable and she may have difficulty releasing urine. She may also be quite irritable. For deficient Kidney Qi consider Jin Gui Shen Qi Wan (Kidney Qi Pill from the Golden Cabinet) and UB 23 Shenshu (Kidney Transporter), Du 4 Mingmen (Gate of Destiny), UB 63 Jinmen (Golden Gate), Ki 3 Taixi (Supreme Stream), Ki 7 Fuliu (Returning Current), and Du 20 Baihui (Hundred Convergences). Spleen Qi may descend and the fetus may drop, compounding the discomfort. Here Bu Zhong Yi Qi Tang (Tonify the Middle and Augment the Qi Decoction) can help as well as UB 20 Pishu (Spleen's Hollow), Du 20 Baihui (Hundred Convergences), St 36 Zusanli (Leg Three Miles), and UB 28 Pangguangshu (Bladder's Hollow). Yi Qi Dao Ni Tang (Benefit Qi and Guide Rebellion Decoction) (Dang Shen (codonopsis), Bai Zhu (atractylodes), Bian Dou (white hyacinth bean), Fu Ling (poria), Sheng Ma (cimicifuga), Jie Geng (platycodon),

Wu Yao (lindera root), Gui Zhi (cinnamon twig), and Tong Cao (tetrapanax)) and Yi Qi Li Shi Tang (Benefit Qi and Disinhibit Dampness Decoction) (Huang Qi (astragalus), Sheng Ma (cimicifuga), Tong Cao (tetrapanax), Gui Zhi (cinnamon twig), Dang Shen (codonopsis), Che Qian Cao (plaintain), Dang Gui (angelica), Wu Yao (lindera root), Ze Xie (alisma), Bai Zhu (atractylodes), and Gu Ya (rice sprouts) may also be helpful. When Damp Heat in the Urinary Bladder presents, use UB 22 Sanjiaoshu (Triple Burner's Hollow), UB 28 Pangguangshu (Bladder's Hollow), UB 32 Ciliao (Second Crevice), UB 53 Baohuang (Bladder's Vitals), UB 63 Jinmen (Golden Gate), and Sp 9 Yinlingquan (Yin Mound Spring Foot), as well as Zi Shen Tang (Enrich the Kidneys Decoction) or Huang Bai (phellodendrum), Che Qian Zi (plantago seeds), Zhu Ling (polyporus), Zhi Mu (anemarrhena), Rou Gui (cinnamon bark), Jie Geng (platycodon), Mu Tang (akenia caulis), Fu Ling (poria), and Hua Shi (talcum).

MOTHERS' GUIDELINES FOR THE SIXTH MONTH
Nutrition

- Watch how much you eat at each sitting. Satiate your hunger with smaller meals to avoid indigestion, and include ginger, mint, and more moving spices.
- Drink lots of water; you'll need more hydration.
- Eat fruit like plums and compact fruit like pears and apples.
- Include adequate dairy this month.
- If you are omnivorous, it is suggested that you eat more animal protein this month, especially wild game.

Lifestyle and exercises

- Mobilize your neck and circle the joints of your wrists, elbows, shoulders, hips, knees, and ankles.
- Perform exercises that awaken your tendons. As you inhale, focus your breath out toward your extremities, extend your wrist joints as far as they'll comfortably go, without straining or using force. As you reach their limit, "snap" them back and exhale. Repeat with any other joint or tendon that feels like it needs more energy.

- Light exercise can help move the energy that is building up. If you haven't been exercising daily, this month requires more movement. Walk, cycle, or swim. Perform activities that require light muscular strength, without straining.
- When uncomfortable, try to take pressure off your belly. Use side-lying support pillows. Lie down and open your hips; do standing hip circles and gentle squats to create more room.
- When you experience physical pain, notice your tendency to resist it or avoid it. See if you can move into the sensation and surround it with your consciousness. Does the sensation change with your attention? Notice if it has any message with it.
- Temper any tendency for sensory overload. Don't strain your eyes, mouth, or ears. Moderate how much information you take in, strange environments, or overly unusual tastes.
- Whether you maintain your own nails or allow someone else to, get yourself a manicure and/or pedicure. This isn't just pampering; the nails are a manifestation of the tendons, which are meant to receive more attention this month.
- If you develop a cold, be wary of taking drying antihistamines.
- You may feel yourself more restless, irritable, and vulnerable. This is normal. If you are on the verge of crying, by all means allow yourself to release the tears.

Self-inquiry exercises

- What have you learned about yourself so far during your pregnancy?
- What has been the greatest life lesson your soul has learned thus far in life?
- What are the greatest gifts you can offer your child?
- What qualities do you possess that you fear you may pass on to your child?
- In what areas of your body do you experience stiffness?
- Do you think you have any rigid beliefs that are harmful?
- How could you soften them?
- What causes you any emotional reactivity?
- What triggers the experience of shame or guilt?

- What do you need in order to forgive yourself?
- In what areas of your life do you need more order or discipline?

Ritual space

Create a ritual with a particular theme for you and your baby to get to know one another's original nature. This can involve prayer, meditation, journaling, or body movements that feel sacred and meaningful to you.

- Include objects or photographs that are meaningful to you.
- Light a candle or incense.
- Sing or play music that you think your baby would like.
- How would your baby want you to move your body in concert with his/hers?

CHAPTER 12

Lungs: Lunar Month Seven

Weeks 24–28

Days 169–196

> No form is the great ancestor of matter.
> No sound is the great ancestor of the voice.
> The child of no form is light.
> The grandchild of no form is water.
> All are created from no form.
>
> —*Huai Nan Zi, Chapter 2*

We come from the swirly depths of the dark and mysterious origin, and if we don't lose our sense of awe at the mystery of life, we remain supple. However, we often exchange the mystery for solidification in the land of the "known." During the seventh phase of the soul's earthly life, the sense of personhood is further ossified. As it thinks of itself, it becomes; thus its views, beliefs, and life direction become more and more predictable and are more challenging to alter. Not only is the being defined by its conditioning, it believes it *is* its conditioning. The seventh month of pregnancy, as we might expect, composes the mineral hard bones. Hand Tai Yin Lung controls the exteriorization of the skin and body hair, and this month the Jing of Wood begins to be accepted.

Month six emphasized how the Stomach digests the world. As we consume the stuff of Earth, what's outside becomes enfleshed as our very self. We'll begin this month with the theme presented by St 25 Tianshu (Heaven's Pivot), which both divides Heaven and Earth, and also connects Heaven and Earth through me. Our next interface between self and non-self is welcomed this month as the Lung meridian, which begins where the Stomach channel ends. Hand Tai Yin, which governs the nose, provides another primal *mouth of Qi*. Heaven has already become the virtue of my inherent self, and now, to paraphrase Qi Bo, *Earth in me becomes breath* (or the ability to breathe). The Lungs also oversee the cutaneous regions of the skin and body hair. The epidermis can be viewed as another partition between me and all-that-is-not-me; it can also be seen as the integument that connects me to all that *appears* to not be me. With a flip of a mental switch, I can experience my skin as either separating me from or connecting me to life.

The Lungs are the first organ to appear on the Horary clock, which organizes the proper order established by Heaven. They imply an inner inkling to awaken, stimulating our winged souls to come alive and resonate with the macrocosm, as the energy of life is pumped in and out, infusing us with heavenly Qi. This capacity places the Lung official in the position to direct the Qi. This first position will prepare the baby to direct its Qi to accept the breath of life to finalize the birthing process. The Lungs house the Po souls through which we are able to touch into and feel the texture of life. The Po impart challenges to the Jing, and as the Lungs direct the Qi, we achieve the ability to rectify our experiences as we move through life. These wings of the Heart descend to fan the Kidney's production of bone and teeth, and also diffuse to the surface to continue to fashion the skin and body hair.

During the auspicious month of seven, the canopy of the Lungs unfurls to reveal the stars, which open the seven orifices to absorb the light of the celestial bodies. This can be seen in two ways, outside in and inside out. We already know that the heavenly realms oversee prenatal creation as the celestial bodies rotate centripetally around the polestar of the developing being. Next, we know that together, the eyes, ears, nose, mouth, skin, and Heart begin to impart a sensory experience of the world to the baby. As the growing being receives sensory input, it also reacts to mom's emotions and moods. It literally experiences how she perceives the world. And if mom is sensitive, she can respond to the state of her baby as well, who, after all, has the whole cosmos behind her. Mom doesn't worry alone; the baby and the Celestial Qi worry with her. Heaven imparts the sensory orifices, which are continuous with the vibratory sensations they convey. They, in turn, are not separate from the internal chemical symphony by which mom perceives reality; she is intimately connected to the world, which is part of heaven...you get it. The microcosm is the macrocosm. The interface between Heaven and me is my original face. I am in the universe that is also within me; Nuwa's face is mine and mine is hers.

The baby obviously doesn't weep when the mother watches a sad movie, as if it, too, was reacting to the tragic plot line. But it is being conditioned by the Heart's ability to perceive the whole. Whatever metaphor we use to describe our "true face" or the "music of the spheres," it can't be perceived like the other senses, nor explained adequately with language. The presence of the divine is so close there is no individual faculty for experiencing it directly. Its vast love and power may be hidden, but never absent. Yet the Heart can directly perceive it when we close our other windows of perception that are being programmed by the stars this month.

The *Huai Nan Zi* describes how the Quintessential Spirit that we receive from Heaven becomes the physical body provided by Earth... *In this way the physical body is completed and the five orbs (spheres of vital energy) are formed... (which parallel the clouds, air, wind, rain and thunder)... The ears and eyes are the sun and moon; the blood and vital energy are the wind and rain...*

Chapter 11 of the *Tao Te Ching (Book of the Way)* reminds us that whether it's the spokes of a wheel, a clay pot, or the space of a room, it's the emptiness that gives things their utility. The same is true of a human being. Our greatest treasure isn't what fills us, but what's there when we're emptied. The soul dances out of emptiness and wraps itself in nature to achieve form. Recall that the flesh fills in around the Stomach tube to create the body structure; similarly, surrounding the orifices that let in food, air, sound, and light, the flesh and bones fill in around the openings to make a face. The bones shape themselves around the bone holes to allow for the orbs and passage of the bundles of firing Qi the *Huai Nan Zi* refers to as *conduits and connections*, which we call nerves. Qi precedes formation, which is then made more solid. If we could separate it, which we can't, Spirit would be first, Qi second, Blood third. The fourth and fifth months provide the Qi and Blood from which the sixth and seventh months derive their muscular force and skeletal strength.

Water Jing imparts our constitutional makeup; Fire Jing furnishes the ability to know and trust ourselves; and Metal Jing imparts order. The fourth agent, Wood Jing, becomes active this month to bestow strength and direction, like the power that causes the seedling to break through the ground and reach toward the sky. The baby receives the essence of Wood in the seventh month in order to help strengthen and solidify the bones. As the essential Qi of Wood goes into the bones and teeth, the marrow takes over red blood cell production. Any disruption here could cause structural or dental problems in the baby, or its teething could be delayed. The rigidity that makes bones and teeth hard is tempered by the softening quality provided by Wood, compassion.

What a journey we have been on thus far! To be the whole of existence in a helpless human form completely vulnerable and dependent for its survival—it takes a mighty force to hold these opposites! Fortunately, we have one. We are human—our heads are in the image of Heaven and our feet the Earth—we are total contradictions and meant to hold paradox. Life isn't meant to make sense, to be all Yin or Yang. As vast space makes up the particles in the atoms in our DNA, we come from nothing and we are simultaneously everything and our little ole' selves all in one bundle. In the great timeless eternity of the ever-present now, Metal holds the past, and Wood faces the future. In the realm where Po and Hun interact, these two ghosts are responsible for the appearance of time. Metal Jing entered last month; Wood Jing this month. Each, as we have described, holds a component of the psyche—the challenges of our curriculum, and their resolution. And we are prepared in utero for these upcoming challenges.

Metal and Fire are in a constant struggle in the chest; as Metal fights for survival, Fire longs for exchange. Metal can insult Fire, controls Wood, and can prevent the Pericardium from full expression.

The Hun and the Po come together in the center where chaos is perfectly resolved. Yet if we don't presently possess the resources to deal with our emotional injuries, they can challenge the primary channels, so the body creates collaterals as temporary holding ditches so we can get on with life. Just like the Luo vessels were created in the fourth month to deal with Blood issues, divergent channels are being created this month to deal with conflicts in the Qi that will most certainly arise as we attempt to rectify our walk of life. These might show up later in life as chronic inflammatory or autoimmune diseases that arise as a fundamental confusion of Wei Qi.

We've talked about the irreducible quality of being ourselves. While it can't be captured by any of the roles we've taken on, there is something so *me* about me that is as challenging to explain as Yuan Qi, but is known by Heart. This inner resource, held within every cell, is what the immune system protects. When Wei Qi is robust and can discern healthy self from non-self, any harmful factor will be neutralized and harmony restored. If, however, we don't have the resources to deal with and expel the deleterious agent, which may be an external pathogen or an emotional injury, the body will utilize Jing, Blood, or Jin/Ye fluids as a medium to hold the pathogen/Wei Qi conflict at bay in these adaptive divergent channels until we either have the Qi and Blood to deal with it, or we no longer have the resources to keep it suppressed. As our Jing, Qi, and Blood decline or are stressed, the dormant evil Qi can seep out and flare up, unleashing symptoms we associate with autoimmune disorders.

Certain conditions can become dormant during pregnancy. Jing is a dense medium for holding latency, and now the Jing is being retained by the fetus. As the divergent channels are being constructed this month, any overwhelm might cause the mother to experience symptoms like achey joints, or may be transmitted to the baby, who could develop arthritic or other reactive conditions.

As Wood Jing enters, so will its Yang characteristics, like working hard and taking charge. This is the month to bring forth motivation and inspiration. Activate any dormant goals and visions that need follow-through. Wood thrives on competition, adaptability, and flexibility. The mother is advised to make flexion and extension movements this month (like lifting light weights) to feel a sense of physical accomplishment, and help facilitate transport of Qi and Blood to the developing skeletal structure. In the sixth month, her musculature was more active; in the seventh month, the tendinous attachments will help to strengthen the bones.

In the seventh month of fetal life, the Lung energies help establish order by hardening the bones and teeth. With so much energy required to travel into the bones, teeth, and divergent channels, Yin Wei and Yin Qiao step in to gather the Yin to help finalize the bone matrix and teeth and fix the required hardness in place. Similarly, during the seventh stage of life, Metal holds our hardened fixations in place. Our acquired conditioning solidifies, and fixations can turn to stasis as we lose the ability to step outside of ourselves and recognize our part in the healing process. Our resources may weaken, and conflicts within the Wei Qi and divergent channels may be unleashed within the system. This does not mean look for pathology to medicate, but perhaps be aware of any rigid holding patterns within so they can be softened. Pay attention to any defensive postures like jaw clenching, shoulder or neck tension, and gently facilitate their release. There will always be something precious underneath.

The baby is vigorously moving around now, tumbling and kicking in response to sounds and touch. It begins to blink. The baby's skin is becoming less translucent, and its sebaceous glands produce a greasy white coating (vernix caseosa) that begins to cover the delicate skin, protecting it from roughening through exposure to amnionic fluid. The lungs produce pneumocytes, which will allow some of the gas-exchanging portions of the lungs to begin exercising their future respiratory function. During weeks 24 to 28, increased fetal breathing activity is noticed. As baby "breathes" in amniotic fluid, it may start to hiccup as the diaphragm responds to the movement through the lungs.

Caring for the seventh month

Because we are starting to pivot toward the third trimester, we will want to include Ki 9 Zhubin (Guest House) with our treatments to help clear any residual toxins during this transitional period, along with mild superficial stimulation of Ren 4 Guanyuan (Origin Pass). The treatment principles that dominate this month are to warm the interior, rid internal Damp and Cold, and strengthen the bones. You may employ UB 11 Dazhu (Great Shuttle), Long Gu (dragon bone) and Mu Li (oyster shell), and bone-strengthening herbs like Xu Duan (dipsacus) and Du Zhong (eucommia). The bones are also particularly susceptible to Dampness, so check the tongue for excess coating.

Because the Lungs are descending to the Kidneys to create the bones, and diffusing to the surface to create the skin and body hair, any type of imbalanced Qi can show up with cold limbs—especially cold hands and feet, as the Lung Qi isn't fully able to reach the exterior. The mother may have shortness of breath, and a feverish sensation. She may crave cold food and drinks, even though she has cold limbs. She should avoid frightening experiences that create emotional cold. Fear's contractile quality can also cause cold hands and feet. If cold limbs are accompanied by shortness of breath and abdominal fullness/chest oppression, Cong Bai (scallions) are the principle herb, which is suggested in tincture form. Cong Bai Tang (Scallion White Decoction) uses 24 stalks of Cong Bai, with Dang Gui (angelica), Huang Qi (astragalus), and Ban Xia (pinellia) to rid internal Damp and Cold. E Guan Shi or Chong Ru Shi (stalactite) are formed in cold caverns, and thus treat a restless fetus with coldness of the limbs. The calcium carbonate helps to warm and draw heat to the exterior. The Yang is going into the bones, and if it can't be tempered, a steaming bone disorder can develop. If the body lacks the Yang it needs, the bones can steam up trying to produce more Heat. The development of Xiao Ke (a wasting and thirsting disorder) can be associated with this pattern. As mom's body tries to retain water in an attempt to regulate body temperature, edema may result.

Pulses should be full, firm, and powerful this month. Continue to support Qi, Blood, and Yang, and provide treatments to keep them moving. Mom should not be given astringents, which will slow things down. Mai Men Dong (ophiopogon), Ren Shen (ginseng), Dang Gui (angelica), Ban Xia (pinellia), and Sheng Jiang (ginger) are all encouraged. She can eat spicy foods to keep Qi and Blood circulating. If there is a weakness in the Wei Qi and divergent channels are already overwhelmed, she may develop autoimmune-type reactivity. Tonify the Qi with Ren Shen (ginseng) or Huang Qi (astragalus) if weak, but watch out for the development of Heat, Dampness, or stasis. Since skin and body hair are emphasized this month, supplement treatments with light massages. Mom is to stay away from damp environments, remain dry, and avoid cold food and drink. Cold in the Stomach prevents the Qi rising to the chest to support the Lung.

Last month we encouraged the tendency toward vulnerability, but this month we need more strength on every level. It would be good to steer clear of sad or tearful topics, because excessive crying will not only strain the mother's Lungs but may also make the fetus restless from overwhelming emotions. Mom would do well to shy away from excessive talking and gossip, which can damage the Lungs. We want to temper the Lungs, but without smothering them. She should stay warm, but avoid wearing heavy clothing, going to saunas, or using hot tubs. The Lungs need to be open and aerated. Excessive sadness condenses energy in the center until its vitality is exhausted. This can tighten the Heart and contract the Yin organs. As the Liver tries to unbind itself, Heat and agitation are produced, injuring the Hun, and zapping imagination and joy. This type of Heat can impact the Pericardium and its relationship with the Bao, transmitting a state of despair and lack of Heat. UB 10 Tianzhu (Celestial Pillar) helps to irrigate the Jin and Ye, and focusing on the quiet joy of the Heart can gently move out sadness.

Liver imbalances can cause counter-currents of Yang Qi, causing mom to develop nosebleeds or Blood-deficient muscular spasms, similar to growing pains. Tonify the Blood and clear excess Yang Qi from the upper body.

In the latter half of pregnancy, along with increased blood volume, progesterone and relaxin soften the smooth muscles in blood vessels, which, along with increased pelvic pressure, can hinder venous return, thus varicosities are common. Check for Luo vessels, and make sure there is adequate Blood before you facilitate their release. Hemorrhoids may also develop, for which UB 40 Weizhong (Supporting Middle), UB 57 Chengshan (Mountain Support), St 36 Zusanli (Leg Three Miles), Ki 3 Taixi (Supreme Stream), and Du 1 Pomen (Long Strong) might be appropriate. Tonify Qi and Blood and lift the Spleen. Long Yan Rou (longan), a major ingredient of Gui Pi Tang (Restoring the Spleen Decoction), contains rutin, which strengthens capillary walls and improves circulation.

Placental damage and intrauterine growth restriction

Intrauterine growth restriction (IUGR) is a condition when the baby's growth is delayed, putting it at risk for health concerns during pregnancy, delivery, and after birth. Failure of the fetus to grow is associated with Qi, Blood, and Yang Vacuity.

Zi Xuan means child suspension. Beginning in the second trimester, it may feel as if something is suspended from the chest cavity below the Heart and diaphragm. As the baby pushes against the chest, symptoms of insomnia, irritability, and anxiety may accompany the discomfort. This can indicate placental insufficiency, or the umbilical cord may be kinked or wrapped around the baby, though these conditions are often asymptomatic. Palpate around Ren 15 Jiuwei (Turtledove Tail) for Luo, and if the mother gets flushed, it indicates rebellious Qi is coming up to the Heart. Massaging the mother can relax the baby and the umbilical cord. Moxa any cold, stagnant areas, perform Tui Na on the back and shoulders, and Gua Sha around the intercostal and diaphragm area. She may also experience back pain—tonify the Kidneys with Xu Duan (dipsacus), Du Zhong (eucommia), and Du Huo (pubescent angelica root) along with her presenting pattern—often Qi and Blood vacuity—for which Ba Zhen Tang (Eight Treasure Decoction) is appropriate. Other potential formulas include:

- Yu Tai Jian Zi Tang (Nurture the Fetus Construct the Child Decoction): Tu Si Zi (cuscuta), Dang Shen (codonopsis), Bai Zhu (atractylodes), Fu Ling (poria), Zhi Gan Cao (prepared licorice), Dang Gui (angelica), Chuan Xiong (cnidium), Shu Di Huang (rehmannia), Bai Shao (white peony).
- Bu Pi An Tai Yin (Great Tonifying the Yin Pill): Dang Shen (codonopsis), Huang Qi (astragalus), Dang Gui (angelica), Bai Zhu (atractylodes), Fu Shen (poria root), Tu Si Zi (cuscuta), Shan Zhu Yu (cornus), Suan Zao

Ren (zizyphus), Shen Qu (medicated leaven), Sheng Jiang (ginger), Da Zao (Chinese date).

- If accompanied by breathlessness and chest oppression, add Xing Ren (apricot seed) and Huo Po (magnolia).
- If Spleen Qi is sunken, prescribe Bu Zhong Yi Qi Tang (Tonify the Middle and Augment the Qi Decoction), use Sp 4 Gongsun (Grandfather-Grandson), St 36 Zusanli (Leg Three Miles), and Du 20 Baihui (Hundred Convergences). If pelvic heaviness accompanies, consolidate Dai Mai with GB 41 Zulinqi (Foot Governor of Tears), and address any sensitive Dai Mai points (GB 26 Daimai (Girdle Vessel), GB 27 Wushu (Five Pivots), and GB 28 Weidao (Linking Path)), perhaps along with superficial needling of Tituo.

Edema of pregnancy—Zi Zhong

As pregnancy progresses, fluid may accumulate in the feet and ankles. The body is producing about 50% more blood and body fluids, and the rapid growth of the fetus has a tendency to obstruct the Qi passing to the lower extremity. Swelling tends to be exacerbated later in the day, the more the mother is on her feet, and during hotter weather. The lack of circulation causes congested tissues. Patterns associated with fluid retention may be due to Damp accumulation from weak Spleen and/or Kidney Yang, or exhausted Yin. The older the woman is, the more likely it will be due to Yin deficiency; the younger she is, it is more likely due to Damp accumulation. Kidney and Spleen Yang are being harnessed to create the baby, leaving less to move and metabolize fluids. If mom's Yang is already weak, it will tax her ability even more. If she develops foot cramps, these relate more to Blood stasis. She should be encouraged to get off her feet and keep them elevated as much as possible, and employ the foot-pumping motion. She can also soak them in a cool (not cold) Epsom salt bath.

SJ 6 Zhigou (Branching Ditch) can help regulate fluid buildup in the Lower Jiao—UB 20 Pishu (Spleen's Hollow), Ren 9 Shuifen (Water Separation), Ren 11 Jianli (Interior Strengthening), Ren 12 Zhongwan (Middle Epigastrium) (massage or very superficial needling), St 36 Zusanli (Leg Three Miles), Sp 3 Taibai (Supreme White), Ki 7 Fuliu (Returning Current), St 21 Liangmen (Beam Gate), and UB 22 Sanjiaoshu (Triple Burner's Hollow) are also options. If her Spleen is weak, use Yi Chi Ren (black cardamom seeds) to build up the Kidney and Spleen Yang, along with Shen Ling Bai Zhu San (Ginseng, Poria, and Atractylodes

Macrocephala Powder). If edema is severe and accompanied by urinary retention, add Ze Xie (water plantain). If breathlessness and chest oppression, add Xing Ren (armeniacae) and Huo Po (magnolia). Another suggested formulation is Li Yu Tang (Disinhibit Constraint Decoction), whose main ingredient is carp, which resolves edema and tonifies Spleen. Add Bai Zhu (atractylodes), Fu Ling (poria), Dang Gui (angelica), Bai Shao (white peony), and Sheng Jiang (ginger). When Kidney Yang is deficient, needle or Moxa UB 23 Shenshu (Kidney Transporter), Du 4 Mingmen (Gate of Destiny), Ki 7 Fuliu (Returning Current), and St 20 Chengman (Assuming Fullness). Zhen Wu Tang (True Warrior Decoction) consists of Fu Zi (wolfsbane), Bai Zhu (atractylodes), Fu Ling (poria), Bai Shao (white peony), and Sheng Jiang (ginger).

MOTHERS' GUIDELINES FOR THE SEVENTH MONTH
Nutrition

- Continue to hydrate and consume enough fiber to avoid constipation.
- Eat glutinous grains like sticky rice and wheat.
- Fish oil and ghee support cholesterol and hormone production.
- Avoid cold foods and beverages. Consume very little raw vegetables like cucumbers and celery. Sauté or simmer your vegetables; even juiced vegetables are energetically "cold."
- Consume calcium-rich foods like sardines and canned salmon with bones in, beans, peas, lentils, edamame, leafy greens, amaranth, almonds and Brazil nuts, seeds like chia, pumpkin and flax, eggs, and bone broth.
- Add more spices to your cooking like scallions, ginger, and peppers, to keep things moving.

Lifestyle and exercises

- Reduce excess activity. Get plenty of rest, but don't become sedentary.
- Skin and body hair are emphasized this month; get light massages or facial massages.
- Dry skin brushing in light motions stimulates the skin, but not too strong or it will have a depleting effect.

- Immerse your skin in different textures—wear soft clothing—feel silk, cashmere, Angora, bamboo; try some essential oils but stay away from heavily perfumed lotions and body oils that might be too much for the delicate nose and skin.
- Get out of your head and immerse yourself in your senses as much as you can. Put your awareness into your fingertips as you feel the fabric you are sitting on. Awaken the sense of sight, smell, and taste, and attend to how your environment stimulates your senses.
- Pay special attention to your teeth this month. Make sure you have enough calcium. If your teeth are weak or sensitive, use natural remineralizing toothpaste or mouthwash.
- Epsom salt foot soaks or baths can help prevent fluid accumulation.
- Avoid cold, windy, or damp environments; stay dry with a dehumidifier if necessary.
- Avoid sad or scary movies or frightening experiences to temper your emotions.
- Go out on a clear night star gazing to absorb the starlight from the night sky.
- Physical movements this month require flexion and extension to strengthen the bones. Lift light to moderate weights—never to the point of exhaustion or requiring you to hold your breath or grunt.
- When you first wake up in the morning, take a few deep breaths, and slowly scan your body from the crown of your head down to your shoulders, your torso, your hips, knees, feet, and reflect on how you feel, how far you've come, and what you and your baby need most to feel nourished today. It could be in the physical, emotional, or spiritual realm.
- Throughout your day, pause, put a hand on the center of your chest and ask, "What do I need?" The more you do this, the more natural it starts to feel. Put another hand on your belly and ask, "What do you need?"
- Smile regularly, first to yourself, and then to your baby. See if you can feel your baby smiling back from within.
- Spend some time sensing what your baby might be experiencing. Convey your understanding internally through your heart, and externally through your touch.

Self-inquiry exercises

- Where are your energies bound up in judgment?
- What dormant projects need to be finished?
- Are there any goals you could reinvigorate?
- What makes you feel like a winner?
- In what areas of your life can you practice more compassion—for yourself or others?
- Continue to attend to the sensations in your body. Move into any pain and discomfort rather than away from it. Learn to read the messages of your body. Surround every sensation with your attention. What are the unique colors, textures, temperatures, or particular messages each physical impression carries?

CHAPTER 13

Third Trimester—
Hun (Wood)

THE TWO GIVE BIRTH TO THE THREE

The god of the southern sea was called Swift, and the god of the northern sea was referred to as Sudden. Between them was the goddess of the center realm, wild and untamed, called Hundun (chaos). Without borders, without boundaries; since there was no particular thing that she was, there was no thing she was not. Swift and Sudden would often meet in the center realm where chaos resided. Hundun would host them with great courtesy, receiving them exactly as they were. Swift and Sudden, moved by Hundun's hospitality, made a plan to return her generosity. "All humans have seven orifices," they said, "so that they can see and hear, eat and breathe. Hundun alone has none. Why don't we bore these for her?" So Hundun graciously received their gifts like she received everything. Every day, for seven days, they bore one orifice in her infinite realm, and on the seventh day, Hundun died.

—Adapted from Zhuang Zi's Inner Chapters, with a goddess spin

Chaos, the cloud of pure potential, appears completely random and disordered because she foreshadows the underlying organizational patterns through which manifestations spontaneously arise. Because she precedes duality, the wild goddess is unpredictable; she doesn't take sides by calling one thing good and another bad. Content with life's unfolding, she can be a true force for change. Giving birth invites us to surrender to chaos. We have very little control over the process. We may live; we may not. We may bring forth a healthy child; we may not.

Only sensate beings experience the dualistic world of time and space, but there is a great price to pay for our finitude. Infinity, as we know it, is sacrificed in the process. While we are created in the image of the mysterious origin and mirror her creation, most of us lose the direct experience of this fact. We believe we *are* the orifices that peer into the world rather than its infinite counterpart. Instead of perceiving what is, our individual karmic tendencies overlay reality with our opinions of what should be, calling situations good or bad; being attracted toward some, resisting others. And we become ever limited as our viewpoints accumulate.

When the Windows of Heaven open we awaken to see we never actually lost our true nature; by a sleight of Shang Di's hand, we only appeared to have left it behind. Whenever we become so accomplished at something that we come to realize it, it loses its tangibility, recedes into the background, and basically inhabits us. We have *captured the soul* of the thing. In the same way, we overlook our most innate property and take our most tangible but illusory attributes to be factual. Our souls seem to be captured in a body, birthed as a character separate from its environment who lives in space and time, lives a certain number of years, becomes defined by life experiences, and dies. The irony of our story is that Hundun could never die; nor, of course, can we.

The Hun give us awareness of our eternal nature; they rise in the mist toward ethereal possibilities of what might possibly become, perceiving a potential future that then initiates a sense of time. In the final act of our creation story, the Hun establish how life's lesson plan, established by Shen, is to be carried out, and the tempo by which the upcoming curriculum will be met. The expression of time will play out moment to moment as the smooth flow of Qi unfolds this life story. The environment in utero will finish programming the fetus' emerging consciousness. Exposed to the weather of its amniotic internal world it will be further imprinted with unique markings like the rings of a tree, receiving the completion of creation's finishing touches. Then, at a predetermined schedule, the rhythmic pulsing of labor will herald the death of its fetal self in the dark womb of its Mysterious Mother, and it will emerge into the cadence of the world, a child.

Will it learn its lessons and achieve its destiny? At the end of its days, will it look back and know that every step of its dance with its Po souls was necessary?

Did it dare go into the darkness of its own underbelly until the light moved within, look its shadows in the face, and rise above every perceived limitation? Did it find the hidden motivations of its most cherished but incorrect assumptions, that in order to be loved others must approve of it, that it somehow wasn't divine in origin so it had to pretend to be something it wasn't? Did it melt out the impure aberrant faculties that corrupted the blueprint of its life to find the unitive principle it was here to discover within? Did it give itself completely to the life it had, holding nothing back in order to find its ultimate purpose where it could serve life most fully? Did it abandon itself to its own heavenly radiance? Did you?

> Every (wo)man is two (wo)men:
> one is awake in the darkness,
> the other asleep in the light.

> —*Kahlil Gibran, Sand and Foam: A Book of Aphorisms*

Human beings, between Heaven and Earth, have the power to bring the light into the darkness and the darkness into the light. This is both an active and passive process, here with the emphasis on the latter. *The secret of the receptive*, which *must be sought in stillness*, allows an influx of Yin power that initiates the Yang outflow.

The immensity of this Yin power has been shut off, and it is time to reclaim it. Sometimes our greatest task is to refrain from initiating movement before its time. Filled with the magnitude of our divine power, we have the force of geysers. Without the Yin at our backs, however, we become weak and passive recipients of intervention (like caesarean sections), attempting to force the external Yang movement. There are all kinds of consequences for this. One of the reasons we've lost our power is that we don't know how to work with the forces within; thus we fear them.

Here's a little recap before we clear the Way.

The Po reigned over the first semester as the physical vehicle was being constructed, providing the raw material for the soul's curriculum through our animal spirits. The genetic potential for survival was programmed into the Jing in the lower Dan Tien, establishing relationship with the past and identification with the body. During the second semester, Shen establishes the epigenetic conditioning we'll encounter, through which our environments become embodied. In the middle Dan Tien, Zong Qi implements our unique temperament and behavioral tendencies that set the stage for how our original blueprint will come up against relational and societal challenges that determine how we'll become identified with the mind and emotions.

Now we enter the third trimester, where the upper Dan Tien will be programmed by the movement of the heavenly bodies to determine how the curriculum will be carried out, moment by moment. This spiritual force is provided by the Hun, the three rarefied aspects of the spirit that provide the ability to envision new potentials as well as the strength to realize them. The Hun provide a connectivity beyond ego communication, which links up the small and supposed separate self with a truer, more expansive sense of ourselves where we have access to eternity and imaginal realms. Associated with Wood and residing in the Liver, the Hun provide movement for the Shen in time. Seen as wandering and swirling activities of the psyche, these three gentlemen allow us to measure the movement of time, penetrate new possibilities, establish goals and plans, and expand into different realities. They will direct the timing of how we will differentiate ourselves in order to become the full beings we were intended to be.

Whether we are coming up against the confines of the uterine wall, or a worn-out identity, Wood, like its emotion anger, is a powerful catalyst of transformation with the capacity to break us free from our bondage. Like its pictograms showing a fish breaking through water tension to transform into a bird in flight, and a slave woman under a man's hand, this impetuous movement is necessary to overcome resistance to evolutionary advancement. Life is a series of attempts to define ourselves and then break out of our confinements as we become more and more alive. A fetus breaks free from the uterus to become a child, who moves into adulthood through the force of being a teenager. Wood is all about the process of emergence, where previous conditioning is moved beyond. When these proper transformative movements toward becoming aren't allowed, stagnation occurs. But all transformations involve encountering the discomfort of our contractions.

What we transform belongs to the realm of Metal, and first we must surrender these confining energies that have been implanted in the first trimester and further conditioned during the second. The hidden jewels of the Po souls, buried like coal in the deep black of the soul, provide fuel for the journey as the

Hun interact with these diamonds in the rough. As the baby comes up against the confines of the uterus, the mother can come up against the limitations of her ego, and if she dares explore and overcome them, this will facilitate the ease of her accouchement.

> What you see outside is what is inside of you.
> And what is inside of you is what is outside of you.
> It is visible and it is your garment.
> If you bring forth what is within you,
> what you bring forth will save you.
> If you do not bring forth what is within you,
> what you do not bring forth will destroy you.
>
> —Elaine Pagels, *Gospel of Thomas*, verse 20, *Gnostic Gospels*

The phantoms that make up the ego are both positive and negative. No matter how rosy our upbringing, no one escapes the internal trauma caused by growing up in this world. We each carry inadequacies we perceive as negative; however, we usually compensate for our perceived inadequacies with a less negative force. These comparatively "positive" compensations also possess the power to distort our perception, keeping us stuck in separation, fearfully competing for our survival: the typical, though outdated, mode of the modern ego. But few of us know how to release our less than healthy psychic contributions to the ancestral line. Associated with the past, the Po tend to replay our most compelling tragedies, reinforcing our identification with them. The poor Po become stuck and can't depart—mostly because they are feared, misunderstood, and corrupted through neglect.

Since we don't know what to do with enemies that live within, we disown and reject them; the Hun project them outside of us, and the Qi that invokes transformation gets locked up, usually around the diaphragm. No matter how difficult it is, we have to face this process—for pain is the price of extracting the old programming so the new can emerge. Giving birth and growing souls requires us to break through limitations. Yet it hurts to relinquish control. It's hard to surrender to what we fear. But until we do, we live in the dimension of trying to control the old to maintain the status quo, remaining stuck in fear of our childhood stress, which, of course, we pass on.

The three Hun interact with our base Po instincts and report our karmic deeds back to Heaven, where our actions are imprinted in the ethereal realm. Each one relates to a Dan Tien, composing the spirit of our intelligence, consciousness, and life force:

- The Hun of the upper Dan Tien is the Bright Spirit or Great Light of the intellect. It allows us to imagine, set goals, use our imaginative powers, and act decisively. This most Yang force of the mind was most revered for the high knowledge it conveyed. This isn't referring to scholarly collection of memorized data, but represents a mind clear of cluttered thoughts, receptive to intuitive guidance from universal intelligence.
- The middle Dan Tien is occupied by the Pleasant Soul, which provides the movement of attraction and desire, the things that give us pleasure or a sense of comfort. This is the connective, relational, and feeling center of the Heart, which also needs to be clear of emotional baggage and defensiveness that obstructs the Pericardium.
- The lower Dan Tien carries the Light of the Fetus, the hidden potential of our life force, producing the impulse to live and the drive that thrusts us toward greater possibilities. Again, cleared of the contraction of personal fear-driven urges that only take self into account, we have access to the collective force behind us.

We could say that our souls live as a spectrum of energy spanning time, space, and dimensionality. Some pretty wild quantum science posits that DNA itself, the foundation of our supposed finite selves, is actually a liquid crystalline substance that receives energetic information from the environment in the form of imagery and archetypes, which is then translated into a three-dimensional holographic image. This energy field organizes and animates matter into a seeming solid reality by what is known as the "phantom effect" (Linda Gadbois, 2018). While this may fly in the face of conventional medical dogma, it certainly resonates with ancient Taoist thought. Just as the Hun report to Heaven and the Po come from the Moon, our souls transmit the heavenly realms into this human dimension. Our egos, being apparitions themselves, do not create. They can only come to the end of themselves, unwrapping our true nature. And who doesn't want that illusion to end?

The more we see and know our failures,
the more by grace we shall long to be filled full of endless joy,
for we are created for that.

—*Julian of Norwich, Revelations of Divine Love*

The spirit or soul of a thing gives it its characteristic power. Humans have long personified the spirits as forces of things unseen: angels, ancestors, legions of demons that disturb the mind, and those that have the power to control us, like Mammon and Bacchus. The Chinese terms Chong, Gu, Gui, and Mo describe the spectrum of unseen evils, like parasitic infections, that have the ability to penetrate our being, causing harm and disrupting our spirit, with Mo being the most malicious. Revisiting the concept from the *Zhubing Yuanhou Lun* (*Origin of the Etiology of Disease*), we each inherit tens of thousands of dispiriting "corpse worms," demonic presences that can be transformed into divine lessons when we hold them in the proper light. Because they infiltrate the body, heart, and mind, these phantom energies might also disturb natural body functions, producing bizarre symptoms. The more we're attuned to our internal terrain, however, we can recognize them, learn their lessons, and allow them to exit.

While Confucianists tried to model behavior to conform to an external system of virtues, Taoist philosophy emphasizes Zi Ran 自然, the natural state of self arising, based upon accepting that things are as they are. Nobody makes moral choices to be bad or unhappy, but we have gotten confused. We haven't been taught the natural laws of life. Positive thinking techniques, like *be kind to yourself*, are like modern-day versions of applying Confucian virtues over a festering psychic wound and don't resolve anything. The Po spirits, lost in the land of an unexamined psyche, can be the source of our internal conflicts that need the Hun's attention so they may be felt and transformed. Yet their Chinese names, like Flying Poison and Stinking Lung, make them difficult to relate to. We can, however, recognize the spirits, unique to each of us, that have become warped, garbling their original survival message. In modern vernacular these hauntings might be likened to the harsh inner critic who rehearses our failures, imprisoning us in a small and circumscribed world where we reconstitute our doubts and self-loathing. They can't leave us alone because we think they're us. The Hun, however, can help escort them to another mind-space where they don't blindly control us. We see them not as us but as an aspect of the collective.

When the distorting spirits are in charge, we feel as if we are possessed. They become part of our hidden identity, rather than a condition of the collective human experience. Many of these emotional patterns stem from early childhood stressors that generated faulty programming, etching patterns so subtle and deep that they feel like a part of our true nature rather than the substance of our false egoic selves. These phantoms love to get us off to ourselves where we feel apart from rather than a part of the pulse of life. As soon as one—say, anger—identifies as "me" (*my* anger), I've just given it the key it needs to access the control panel in the upper realms where it can take over the entire queendom. Xi Wang Mu (Queen Mother of the West) can no longer restore harmony until the lower self relinquishes control, and now the whole apparatus functions at the lower vibration of control that keeps us out of the immortal realms.

While the Po are experienced as bodily sensations, they need the Hun's ability to root in the Liver and open our inner eyes so we can recognize any distortions, and witness any negative power they've had over us. Residual ghostly presences, Gui, can remain attached to the Po and haunt us. Yet as the phantom's mask is exposed, it comes out of hiding and begins to release its hold. Most of these faulty programs are excesses that disguise underlying deficiencies. It can be helpful to identify them according to the energies they contort:

- Those that obstruct the mind and intellect, and represent spiritual greed, ambition, and self-aggrandizement, like the Know It All, keep us locked in our heads.
- Those that corrupt our relational capacity to connect, distort our desire for emotional comfort, or through which we take more than our degree of satiation might be called the Glutton or Sloth; they obstruct the light of the Heart.
- Those that misrepresent our physical impulses might turn into phantoms like the Hoarder or Seductress, which make their home in the lower Dan Tien and obstruct our life force.

There is a divine timing that belongs to the Hun, and there is usually no need to rush this process; when we are ready, the proper environment for the Hun and Po's interaction is given. Gravidity, however, provides a certain urgency to clear the "guest house" of unwanted visitors that may have possessed us with traumatic reactions that violated the constitution. We use Ki 9 Zhubin (Guest

House) between trimesters because it accesses the Hun and Po's meeting place, which is in the Heart. Like Swift and Sudden, the two souls are welcome to mingle here, but not to overstay their welcome. The three Hun and the seven Po are meant to play together, integrating the unfinished pieces of our own brokenness, but they are not meant to have the final say in who we are.

If Gui are ignored, they tend to form a sticky film over our organs and consciousness. The Yang light of Hun helps us not only to recognize them, but also to evaporate the Phlegm that keeps them obscured. The Hun, which follow the Shen and report directly to the Heavenly Emperor, play a role in the intellect, memory, and imagination, and have access to symbolic images from the collective realm through which they can interact directly with the phantom programs. We can use the Hun to recall the origin of the distortions, and apply explicit names that personify them. As we begin to acknowledge them, their Hun counterpart can shine the light of compassion on them so each can reveal the underlying need it is obscuring. When we see that the manipulative Pleaser is masquerading as the need to be loved, we can bring it to the middle Dan Tien, where the Pleasant Soul welcomes it.

When our rejected parts come out and meet Wood's virtue of kindness, they cease to be enemies, caused by our own resistance, and therefore lose their power to haunt us. If we don't begin with acceptance and surrender, however, the Hun can't reach them with the compassion required to loosen the ego's hold, which only knows how to deny or fiercely protect. Yet, if we are devoted to healing, we can relinquish control and encounter some pretty miraculous healing on the other side. We no longer relate to these distortions as *us*. If we can be aware of them, they can't be our true selves; thus we have relinquished the soul of the thing. Their emotional charge exits through the Mysterious Pass, and we are free of their identifying hold. Our biggest lessons are learned most humbly.

As we stop trying to outrun our shadows, our illusory possessors loosen their hold, revealing the true self of whom we can't ever lose possession. The unitive eye of Shen that lives in true freedom has always had the ability to inhabit the darkest night and the brightest light. No longer possessed by the ego's false hold we are back in possession of our authentic self, rooted in Tao. As Lao Tzu's eyebrows sweep away the delusion, our systems miraculously harmonize to the vibration of divine synchrony.

The human soul continues to wrap itself up in emotional attachments as life transpires, locking up these emotional energies at the Blood level, which, if unresolved, remain stuck in lower vibrational planes. These can obscure our intuitive feelings, through which the Wei Qi navigates life. Interesting that we all seem to share the same allegorical issues, as if all of humanity draws from the same pool of psychic representations. Chapter 2 of *Zhuang Zi* speaks of the Hun's ability to commune and relate intimately during sleep. The Hun access the collective unconscious via symbolic images that are a part of the shared human experience and relay them to consciousness during dream states. While Shen belongs to Heaven, Hun are ours, although they follow the spirits. The Hun also help us communicate with one another at another level entirely, where we can literally experience the transparency of one another's souls. Claude Larre contrasts the Hun's ability to commune with other souls against what's considered "normal" communication where we *hurl ourselves at the multiplicity that other beings set to render themselves opaque.* The Hun connect us to our heavenly origin—as a deeper, vaster, more soulful aspect of ourselves pervades the immanency of our dynamic and relational lives.

When an individual leaves the earthly plane, their unresolved issues may wander the earth as a ghostly energy, looking for someone else who vibrates similarly, in whom it might be allowed to take up residence. At death, Taoist priests would call the Hun back, inviting them to reinhabit the body, providing another chance to release any unresolved matter. If the Hun returned, life would continue. If not, the Hun were presumed to return to Heaven (via Du 20 Baihui (Hundred Convergences)) and the Po souls returned to Earth (via Du 1 Pomen (Long Strong)). As we clean up psychically, not only do we correct our physiology; we also scour time and space to find the indissoluble unity of our place in the whole. We banish nothing, while we veritably clear up the collective. Hun connect us to the ethereal plane where everything is in its proper place in our vast, spacious selves, an intrinsic part of the cosmic whole, connected to everything that ever has been, is, or will be, that is, where Hundun reigns supreme.

> My left eye is the sun;
> it belongs to Pangu and lets me take in the world.
> My right eye is the moon;
> it belongs to Nuwa and lets me take in myself.

The celestial bodies rotate around the central eye, which belongs to the Tao.

The Hun souls relate to dreams, imaginings, and the unitive third eye, as they wander the borders of consciousness in the nine Heavens and nine Earths. We are so vast! Whatever we are perceiving, from a knot in consciousness to a star in the sky, we can view our thoughts like heavenly orbs, and be free of them. We are learning to follow our north star where our central core magnetizes the experiences we are meant to have while simultaneously manifesting the gifts imparted by Heaven that long to be expressed in the world. Our true destiny is always contributory to the collective and to the cosmos. We know we are following the Way when our state of being and doing are not separate, when we're in devoted service to that which wants to be born. Expressing the soul's mandate is accompanied by a flow of peace and joy, which effortlessly opens up the next synchronous step on our journey. When we follow the Way, we are always perfectly placed in the exact location where our unique offerings are to be called forth, and the unimaginable is allowed to manifest.

Whether we are birthing the Tao, a new self, or a baby, the rules are the same. The Hun can help us break through bonds of confinement, send us symbolic messages, and set us in the right place at the right time. The final phase of any life process is associated with the function of differentiation—not to become more distinct and separate, but to reintegrate the separate and cut-off parts of ourselves. As we face these most challenging lessons, we actually become more authentic and innocent representations of the whole. Through the upper Dan Tien, we learn to discern and attend only to what resonates with our cosmic purpose. As we come to our finale, we have only so much energy to expend. But we will make the finish line, for hope is the upper Dan Tien's equivalent of the biological urge, which propels us forward with a childlike certainty in our step—not knowing what's going to meet us, but not needing to.

As we move into the third trimester, Qi and Blood stores will be consumed to finalize our reproduction. Life in the womb will become compressed; hormones will surge along with emotions. Energies may stagnate as time seems to stall. Compassion is the key. We will be coming to the end of this journey soon enough and will have to surrender to the unknown so a new possibility can be birthed. All new beginnings are accompanied by new awakenings. This process is meant to expand us out of our old casings and open us to a new view of life and a new vision of ourselves. For the next three months we will bring this vision into being until the soul is ready to emerge. Then we'll venture with the goddesses to invoke the mystery, cleansed of the ego's residual internal conflicts, ready to enter the birthing place of galaxies, holding on to nothing. Hundun's got this.

I go within and close the doors.
Darkness enfolds the matrix of my earthly body.
The particle returns to a wave.
Nothing but consciousness inside and out.
The windows of perception are cleansed; the veil lifts.
Past and future spiral into a light
that rotates according to its own law.
Where am I in this eternal exchange I cannot tell.
The shell cracks.
I give birth to the Tao.

MOTHERS' GUIDELINES ENTERING THE THIRD TRIMESTER
Lifestyle and exercises

- Since planning and nesting are functions of the third trimester, take care not to let any demands overwhelm you. Set aside a certain amount of time each week to make any necessary preparations for the baby and for yourself.
- Ask for any help you need for this.
- Our next task in the third trimester is to practice stillness, cultivating the power of Yin. Spend as much time as you are able basking in the spirit that has brought you this far. Without reading, watching TV, or creating any distraction for yourself, are you able to be internally quiet, in the potent space of waiting?
- Can you feel your baby and yourself held by a force that isn't you but isn't other than you, that has carried the long line of mothers before you to their destination?
- How can you learn to trust and surrender to this force more?

Exorcizing distortions
Since the Qi follows the Mind, cleaning up any residual psychic distortions that obstruct energy flow will help prepare for a smooth transition from gestation to parturition.

- Scan through your body, memory, or emotional banks for your most troubling or trauma-inducing issues. Conscious or not, your baby is marinating in them too.

- Where in your body are they located? They might occupy your thinking and live in the head; they may cause anxiety or a feeling of obstruction in your chest; or they may be held deep within the belly.
- Feel each one at a time, and become familiar with its effects.
- At this point, it may become evasive, and attempt to go into hiding. Be persistent. Spirits want validation, so you can name these phantom energies.
- Provide a description of each energy, giving it a specific or descriptive name. Be imaginative and creative. You have to own it before you can become free of it: The Belittler, The Naysayer…
- What need, fear, or hurt is it camouflaging underneath?
- What has this distorted energy provided for you? How has it protected you?
- When you've acknowledged its role, its lesson, or its gift, can you feel compassion for it?
- Are you willing to let this part of you be healed? If not, can you feel compassion for this part of yourself?
- Can you thank it for its presence and allow its emotional charge to be released?
- Recognize the energy it took to resist or keep this phantom in place, and feel it unwind.
- Think of a symbol or an image in your mind's eye that can represent the gift this phantom energy has brought to you.

Soul inquiry

- Are you beginning to remember what you're here for?
- Can you name at least one attribute of your authentic spirit?
- Are you becoming a different woman from the one who started this journey?
- How?
- What heaviness have you relieved your offspring of thus far?
- Use your imagination in new and expansive ways. Continue to communicate with your baby and see if you can sense different aspects of

their soul, where they've come from, and where their life direction might take them.

- Can you recognize the amazing healing work you're accomplishing?
- Give yourself credit. Gestating souls is the most incredible work a woman can do.

CHAPTER 14

Large Intestine: Lunar Month Eight

Weeks 28–32

Days 197–224

> The Two give birth to the Three,
> and the Three give birth to the ten thousand things.

As we enter the third trimester, we are in the domain of the Liver and the Hun. Most of our care during the rest of the pregnancy will be to prepare for a smooth labor and delivery. Hand Yang Ming will provide the decisive assertion of Yang to the child, and the necessary push to ensure survival from now on.

> In the secret hour of life's midday
> the parabola is reversed,
> death is born...
> Waxing and waning make one curve.
>
> —*Carl Jung, Psychological Reflections*

With reference to pregnancy, life, birth, or death, we can listen to the wisdom of the moon, which oversees the process of embodiment and disintegration. In its movement toward apparent dissolution, our closest celestial body reveals that supposed endings merely provide the Essence needed for renewal. And in the process of turning pregnancy toward birthing, the baby and its mother undergo an inner ripening. We are beginning our descent.

Like all new beginnings, as we transition out of the second and into the third trimester, we begin by releasing all that has come before to prepare for emergence.

During the eighth phase of life we are urged to relinquish all that unnecessarily confines us, and Metal, which governs the eighth lunar month of pregnancy, provides the best opportunity to surrender inflexible holdings from the past. New possibilities arise when we are willing to let go of attachments. In response to this readiness to meet change, a new energy is called in to guide us into the future.

Arm Yang Ming harmonizes the Heart and quiets the breathing. Wood controls Earth, and the final agent, Earth Jing, is accepted this month in order to nourish and fatten the baby up, and provide the integrity needed to complete the composition of the integument. The Essence of all of the elemental agents has been received, but we still have to finalize a few movements before the child will be ready to make its entrance.

This month the baby will become enveloped by the cutaneous regions, Pi Ge 革, that travel to the sensory organs. The Large Intestine directs this movement through its control of the nine orifices, which will be completed this month. The skin matrix is fully functional now; it is covered with hair, and is referred to as Pi Mao 毛. Last month the stars opened up the seven facial orifices to take in the world. As they receive the Qi from Earth, the pure aspect will be sent by the Stomach to the sensory orifices, and then to the perineal area to open the remaining two lower orifices.

As Metal strengthens the instinct for survival, it allows us to both live and let go fully. This dynamic is illustrated as the Large Intestine directs the opening of Po Men at the anal area. This being is fattening up and will soon be surviving on its own, where it will have to do its own releasing. Meanwhile, the walls of its uterine home are closing in. As it becomes more cramped and confined, the baby will soon exercise the need to break out.

The nine orifices are now fully formulated and functional, ready to receive stimulation. Thus the mother is advised to avoid anything overly invigorating to any of her nine orifices. She should remain somewhat reclusive this month, or the child may not be properly balanced. If her senses are overly aroused this month, it can predispose to excess Wind after the umbilical cord is severed.

Cutting the umbilical cord activates the nine orifices. If hyper-arousal causes Wind to enter the child, spasms may present as some type of neurological expression like infantile epilepsy, tetanus, or seizures. SJ 18 Chimai (Spasm Vessel) benefits the orifices and pacifies the Wind that may cause infantile convulsions.

The Yang Qi provided by Yang Ming, which also plays a crucial role in fluid metabolism and distribution, finalizes the activity at the surface layers of the skin this month by tightening the Cou Li. This process nourishes the facial muscles and keeps the skin supple, while transmitting the correct pattern of the fetus' particular skin texture, which will express its identifying features, Li 理.

Later, after five or so cycles of seven, these initial etchings will be magnified by the inevitable depletion of Yang Ming, as well as whatever weathering the being has experienced on its life journey. But this month they are receiving their final touches.

While the Lungs diffuse and descend to bring about release, the Large Intestine provides the heat to finish "cooking" the fetus, while simultaneously moving out waste material. As carbon must be pressurized underground to transform a lump of coal into a diamond, the fetus will begin to glow with its own inner luminosity.

While the initial facial structures came together between the second and third months, now the facial movements become quite complex, conveying expressions like laughing, crying, and scowling. The ever-maturing baby now directly communicates with its environment and exhibits signs of agitation to certain foods, environments, sounds, and ultrasound waves.

As the Shen fully extends itself through the Pi Ge, the baby develops its own auric field of sorts, and it will begin to emanate a light (Gong), which will glow at birth. At least two of the medical APGAR score (appearance, pulse, grimace, activity, and respiration) criteria—appearance and grimace, define this this healthy glow. If the baby doesn't exude this vibrancy of Shen, the imbalance likely occurred in the eighth month.

Caring for the eighth month

While the mother's Qi and Blood have been busy nourishing the fetus, she is likely tired and worn-out. Fortunately, this predisposes her to nature's urgings to remain calm and quiet without too much mental or emotional stimulation so she may conserve her energy for delivery. She will have to eat enough to sustain the Yang Qi, and should remain properly hydrated to support body fluids and Essences.

During the eighth month, our major herb will be Bai Shao (white peony), and Shao Yao Tang (Peony Decoction) to nourish the Blood and Yin, calm Liver Blood and Wind, clear Heat and Toxicity, and move the bowels. We can also employ Ren Shen (ginseng), Sheng Jiang (ginger), Gan Cao (licorice), and Huo Po (magnolia) as needed. Treatment principles will include tonifying the Yin of the Lung and Stomach to nourish the skin, regulate the waterways, and ensure proper hydration. Sang Shen (mulberry), Gou Qi Zi (Chinese wolfberry), and Yu Zhu (polygonatum) make good tonics. The eighth month isn't the time to move the Blood, but to stimulate the Wei Qi level.

The mother's pulse should be big, firm, and full of power, and the moderate level should have adequate Yin. Thready pulses may indicate emerging neurological issues in the child. If you note any tight floating pulses indicating stagnation, you may begin to disinhibit the nine orifices with small amounts of Yuan Zhi (polygala) and Shi Chang Pu (acorus). Larger amounts can be used when we want to facilitate cervical dilation in the tenth month.

We will also begin to prepare to mature the baby and prevent postpartum difficulties. Once the baby's skin, or peel, has been completed, a treatment principle called *ripening the baby* tonifies the Qi and Blood and helps fatten up the baby, so, like ripened fruit, it can easily fall off the tree. Certain herbs are said to make the baby "slippery" so it can slide out at its proper time. Bie Jia (turtle shell) and Dan Shen (salvia) have this effect, which is one of the reasons they are contraindicated during pregnancy. But they can be incorporated during this time to help promote delivery. Sang Shen Fang (Ripen the Baby Formula) consists of Dan Shen (salvia), Dang Gui (angelica), Chuan Xiong (cnidium), Bai Zhu (atractylodes), and Ren Shen (ginseng). Simmer equal amounts of Bei Mu (Sichuan peppers) in pig fat. Make into a paste with the remaining herbs and take one spoonful per day. This will help tonify Qi and Blood, alleviate constipation, and prepare for delivery.

The mother may experience heartburn and reflux after meals. She may also experience general aches and heavy legs. Ren 12 Zhongwan (Middle Epigastrium) may be massaged or needled with a short needle, parallel to the skin. Since we are at a transition month, Pc 6 Neiguan (Inner Pass) and Ki 9 Zhubin (Guest House) are recommended.

As the uterus presses on the bladder and colon, proper elimination may be prevented, resulting in constipation and the build up of toxins. In order to release waste, the Large Intestine has to remain lubricated. Body fluids must flow to the upper orifices and be released through the two lower ones. Since we won't be needling the Large Intestine channel, we may employ Yang Wei and Yang Qiao Mai this month, as well as St 37 Shangjuxu (Upper Great Hollow).

The mother should avoid harsh windy conditions that may exacerbate skin sensitivity. She can also uncover any hidden issues of her Heart she may have missed, allowing them to rise to the surface, while becoming aware of any external resistance she may be harboring and release it. Her pores should be able to close to retain liquids internally or open to relinquish fluids. Because of her susceptibility to Wind and Cold conditions, she should stay inside more this month.

While the baby's external sensitivity increases, a classical symptom the mother may exhibit is skin discomfort with heightened reactivity to touch. She may experience sensations of prickling or like something is crawling over her skin. While Ll 11 Quchi (Crooked Pond) is usually helpful to address skin reactions, we'll avoid needling Arm Yang Ming this month, so some other points you may employ include SJ 5 Waiguan (Outer Pass), Sp 10 Xuehai (Sea of Blood), UB 12 Fengmen (Wind Gate), UB 13 Feishu (Lung's Hollow), UB 17 Geshu (Diaphragm's Hollow), and UB 63 Jinmen (Golden Gate); you may also calm the Spirit and Po with points like Ht 4 Lingdao (Spirit Pathway), Ht 7 Shenmen (Spirit Gate), Lu 3 Tianfu (Heavenly Residence), Lu 7 Lieque (Broken Sequence), and UB 42 Pohu (Po Door).

The Water point of the Heart, Ht 3 Shaohai (Lesser Sea), can be utilized in conjunction with SJ 19 Luxi (Skull's Rest) to lift up the spirit of the child; soon it will lose connection with the mother's Heart, causing the baby to descend.

Obstetric cholestasis

This disorder may develop when the liver and gallbladder become too sluggish to process the high hormones of pregnancy, causing fat toxins to accumulate in the blood. It typically develops during the third trimester, but may begin early in pregnancy. As bile builds up in the liver, the main symptoms are sudden and severe itching, without rash. This condition is treated by addressing the sluggish Liver and Gallbladder: start with GB 31 Fengshi (Wind Market) and SJ 5 Waiguan (Outer Pass), and add Lv 2 Xingjian (Moving Between), Lv 3 Taichong (Great

Surge), Lv 14 Qimen (Cycle Gate), and GB 24 Riyue (Sun and Moon) as needed. In months other than the eighth, also include Ll 11 Quchi (Crooked Pond).

Amniotic fluid abnormalities

The Large Intestine plays a major role in fluid metabolism, especially in the lower burner. Early in pregnancy the fetal lungs contribute to amniotic fluid production. Beginning in the second trimester, as the fetal kidneys produce urine, they are the main source of amniotic fluid for the rest of the pregnancy. The amount of amniotic fluid available, which usually peaks around 36 weeks gestational age, is based on how much fluid is produced and how much is removed from the amniotic sac.

Jin fluid transmits all vital frequencies that support life, and is maintained by regulation of the waterways. Fluid metabolism begins with the origin of fluids, the Stomach, which sends clear fluids to the sensory orifices and to the Spleen for distribution to the rest of the body, which the Lungs then diffuse and disperse, and the Kidneys vaporize. The turbid fluids pass to the Small Intestine—which plunges into the depths and again separates the thin pure fluids from the impure, allowing what, according to its discernment, will enter into the Blood. The Gallbladder separates the pure and turbid associated with irregular fluid physiology via the Curious Fu and Extraordinary Vessels. From the Small Intestine, the pure become body fluids, and the turbid aspect goes on to the Large Intestine, which releases the unnecessary. The intestines recirculate water, and send on to the Urinary Bladder, which stores, provides transformed fluids for the body, and ultimately excretes them. All of these organs must be functioning and communicating optimally to regulate amniotic fluid.

"Oligohydramnios" is a term to describe deficient amniotic fluid, insufficient to meet the demands to cushion the baby, allow for normal movement, and Lung development. Diagnosed by ultrasound, oligohydramnios may be due to maternal, fetal, or placental issues. Anti-inflammatory, angiotensin-converting, and enzyme-inhibiting medications can inhibit blood flow to the fetal kidneys; dehydration and congenital or chromosomal issues that impact proper fetal digestive or renal function can contribute. Loss of fetal movement, referred to as *a dried fetus that is not moving*, may prompt concern, although the condition is often asymptomatic.

Maternal issues may manifest as Yin and or Blood deficiency, and Heat drying fluids and damaging the Blood. Certain studies have found Dan Shen (salvia) and Sheng Di Huang (rehmannia) preparations to be useful.

"Polyhydramnios" describes a scenario where excess amniotic fluid builds up. Associated with fetal abnormalities, Rh incompatability, infections, abruptio placenta, and umbilical cord prolapse, polyhydramnios may cause premature birth. Maternal diabetes mellitus may also cause the fetus to develop hyperglycemia and polyuria, increasing amniotic fluid levels. Focus on proper fluid metabolism, making sure the mother's Kidney and Spleen energies are strong enough, and eliminating any intestinal stagnation.

Abruptio placenta

The placenta can detach from the uterine wall, causing vaginal bleeding, back and abdominal pain, uterine rigidity or contractions, and fetal restlessness. Depending on the severity of separation, this condition can deprive the baby of nutrients and oxygen, and may result in fetal death. While trauma or abdominal injury may lead to placental separation, Chinese medicine considers the causative factor to be Wind causing the placenta to separate, often from an underlying Yin and Blood deficiency, or excess Liver Yang.

Symptoms include vaginal bleeding, and abdominal and back pain in the last twelve weeks of pregnancy. Depending on the degree of placental separation, and how close the baby is to term, treatment may include bed rest or caesarian section. While our treatments throughout pregnancy may be able to prevent placental abruption, in the event it occurs, our treatments should be supportive. Continue to nourish Yin and Blood, and subdue Liver Yang and/or Wind. Many formulas for gestational and postpartum Wind Stroke utilize non-toxic herbal medicines with only one or two ingredients, including Da Dao (glycine), Du Huo (pubescent angelica root), Ge Gen (pueraria), Mai Men Dong (ophiopogan), Gan Cao (licorice), and Sheng Jiang (fresh ginger).

Placenta accreta, on the other hand, is a condition where the placenta adheres too deeply into the uterine lining, making it difficult to separate and expel postpartum. In this case, our treatment principle will be to invigorate stagnant uterine Blood.

Pre-eclampsia

The winds of change are coming. The mother's weight, blood volume, and fluid levels have been dramatically increasing throughout pregnancy, potentially resulting in edema, and increased pressure in the vasculature and Liver, which may be compounded by intestinal stagnation. If these have not been adequately addressed and she begins to feel faint, experience dizziness, headaches, abdominal pain, and blurred vision, they may herald the warning of internal Wind developing into pre-eclampsia.

Pre-eclampsia is a potentially life-threatening disorder of pregnancy where blood pressure spikes (to over 140/90 taken twice or 160/110 once) and protein is dumped in the urine (which may appear turbid or cloudy) and may lead to organ failure. Additional signs and symptoms include shortness of breath caused by fluid collecting in the lungs, elevated liver enzymes, serum creatinine, thrombocytopenia, and potential renal failure. Conventional medical treatment is supportive and includes anti-hypertensives, diuretics, and corticosteroids to hasten fetal lung maturation. Pregnancy-induced hypertension causes changes in the uterus, which can obstruct blood flow to the placenta and develop into eclampsia, from the Greek word for lightning, which indicates the condition has progressed to induce convulsions, and at which point anti-seizure medication is given.

At the initial stages, acupuncture, dietary therapy, and herbal medicine can help to lower blood pressure, clear fluid retention, and stave off eclampsia.

The pulses are often full or wiry, which comes from intestinal stagnation. It is important to make sure the Small Intestine is separating the pure from the turbid and the Large Intestine is eliminating, or toxins can recirculate to the Stomach, which then fails to descend. This can cause the baby to be born with weakened immunity, sensitivities, and allergies. Autointoxication can also stir up Wind that agitates the nervous system. The divergent channels can deposit these Fire toxins into the bones; Moxa Ll 15 Jianyu (Shoulder Bone) and Ll 16 Jugu (Great Bone) to help break up any Qi, Blood, or Phlegm stasis. Make sure the Liver is able to keep up (Lv 2 (Moving Between), Lv 3 (Great Surge)) in order to clear the Blood, or the baby may be born with jaundice. Use Wind points like GB 20 Fengchi (Wind Pool) and Du 16 Fengfu (Wind Mansion), and St 40 Fenglong (Abundant Bulge) for Phlegm.

Magnesium sulfate may help relax the vessels and prevent eclampsia from developing. Open the Yang Qiao vessel with UB 62 Shenmai (Extending Vessel) to address floating Yang. Prior to the onset of Wind, there was likely an underlying deficiency. If Yin is inadequate to carry the baby through pregnancy, it may be unable to anchor the Yang, leading to Liver Yang rising, Liver Blood stasis, and stirring up Wind. Itchy papules may also appear, which can be addressed with GB 31 Fengshi (Wind Market) and SJ 5 Waiguan (Outer Pass).

When Liver Yang rising is the culprit, needle GB 20 Fengchi (Wind Pool), Lv 3 Taichong (Great Surge), and LI 11 Quchi (Crooked Pond) (although not during the eighth month).

For Liver Blood deficiency, needle St 36 Zusanli (Leg Three Miles), Lv 8 Ququan (Spring at the Bend), Lv 3 Taichong (Great Surge), and LI 11 Quchi (Crooked Pond).

For Liver and Kidney Yin deficiency, use UB 23 Shenshu (Kidney Transporter), LI 11 Quchi (Crooked Pond), and Lv 3 Taichong (Great Surge).

Spleen Yang deficiency will benefit from UB 20 Pishu (Spleen's Hollow), Sp 9 Yinlingquan (Yin Mound Spring Foot), and St 36 Zusanli (Leg Three Miles), and with Kidney Yang deficiency add UB 23 Shenshu (Kidney Transporter) and Du 4 Mingmen (Gate of Destiny).

Cannabis and sesame seeds promote the removal of toxins. Use moist laxatives, fats, and oils to calm the nerves. Other popular herbs are Zhu Li (bamboosa) and Gou Teng (gambir); and Ze Xie (alisma) can be used to help release the Bladder. Sun Si Miao was fond of using Zhen Zhu (pearl powder) and minerals to subdue Wind. Shi Jue Ming (abalone shell) is not recommended, however, as it weakens the Liver, which can injure the baby's neurological system. Avoid using Mu Tong (akebia caulkis); it may stimulate milk flow via the Small Intestine, which may give the message to begin the birthing process.

MOTHERS' GUIDELINES FOR THE EIGHTH MONTH
Nutrition

- Remain well hydrated. Have water, coconut water, or water with electrolytes on hand at all times. You don't need to drink a lot at one sitting; it will be important to keep your intestines moving this month.
- No dry foods, preserved fruits, or fried food.
- Avoid bitters, but it is okay to eat spicy food.
- Eat lots of berries—raspberries, blueberries, and blackberries are

great for bowel health. Loganberry, a cross between a raspberry and blackberry, makes a great snack that can strengthen capillary walls and improve circulation to prevent varicose veins.

- Include seeds like sesame and flax to keep the bowels moving.

Lifestyle and exercises

- Avoid wind, severe weather, and drastic changes in your environment.
- Avoid straining the lower abdomen.
- Do not get up too quickly from a sitting or sleeping position; allow yourself to gently rise up.
- Avoid overstimulating the senses. Try to remain calm. Breathe deeply and relax.
- Try not to irritate your skin. You may need to discontinue any lotions, makeup, artificial skin products, or laundry detergents that may irritate your skin this month.
- Elevate and pump your feet to encourage fluid and lymphatic movement.
- Breathe into your belly as much as you are able.
- Continue to strengthen your perineal muscles.
- Put your attention in your belly, buttocks, thighs, and calves.
- Feel your feet connect to the ground.

Self-inquiry exercises

- You already know how to connect to your baby; what are some of the ways you and your baby have been able to communicate with each other?
- Can you encourage and give your baby support for its upcoming entrance?
- How ready do you feel for your baby's arrival?
- What still needs to be done that causes you concern?
- Are you getting adequate help?

CHAPTER 15

Kidney: Lunar Month Nine

Weeks 32–36

Days 225–252

> Every moment life begins all over again.
> Deep within every cell is a force that creates; a force that heals.
> Too mysterious to be given a name,
> the whole earth is pregnant with it.
> If we follow the Tao, completion is inevitable.

Let us return to the Mysterious Mother who birthed the cosmos and yield to her wisdom. She who has guided us this far will not let us go. Herein lies our trust. We have been preparing to surrender to the inevitable. And in order to surrender, we must have trust, a theme exemplified by the Kidneys. The spirits inhabit our physical Essence through the Kidneys, which represent the heroic journey of our arriving fully to this life. There is a challenge in really stepping up to own this life, and the Kidney channel holds the narrative of how we will use our Will to resolve issues around stability, security, stamina, and ambition.

The Kidney channel, which ascends from our feet to the chest, represents the ladder of our destiny. Propelled by the engine of personal Will depicted by the starting point in the feet, as we move out into the world, the sheer effort of willful control can be relinquished and eventually something higher, fed by the deepest part of us, pulls us as if from above. We can trust this movement. While the lotus is initially pushed from the mud, eventually it's all about the flowering. The need to constantly summon our Wills is replaced by following the quiet whispers of the Heart, and choices are made from a different level, although always rooted where we stand. This isn't a direct trajectory upward toward the light—we must swim in and out, spiraling back to our watery depths again and again until we are transformed into birds in flight.

> In the north there is an abyss where the great fish resides.
> This great fish rises up from the sea to become
> the majestic bird which flies straight to the south.

The Kidneys hold the mystery of our watery origin that perpetually flows into life, ensuring continuity of vital circulations through the meridians. In utero, the life force has reached a certain completion and has exteriorized into skin and hair. Now comes an inner compression, which, like fear, heralds the stirrings of new things coming into being. Everything has matured and is in its correct place, and is exhibiting just the right amount of movement. This full development will enable a specific pattern to unfold in the life of the baby.

In the ninth month the *essential Qi of the stone* is received, which represents a concentration of the Essence, assigned to the Kidney official that is in charge of firmness. It provides a certain definition, like the completion of hair and the hardness of bones and teeth that will remain after the life force has gone. The stone also represents the reality of death, like a gravestone, as fetal life comes to an end. As the Large Intestine signifies letting go into the depths of the underground, Metal passes the baked Earth off to Water where the Kidneys provide the pressure that will help Jing solidify and transform into a precious gem, like jade. The fetus must dare to die to life in utero in order to summon the courage of water to emerge.

In the ninth month, the mother *loosens her belt and waits for the right moment,* while patiently, beneath the surface, the Kidney dynamics are being established.

The left and right Kidneys, representing our double-stranded genetic starting point linking us all the way back to the origin, are the first embodiments of duality. As such, the Kidneys hold and blend opposites. Their ability to consolidate into firmness is surrounded by a surrendered softness, characterized by Water. Throughout life, these polarities will provide the tension that will propel it to find its way back to its origin.

In his discourse on "The nature of aging and longevity," Heiner Fruehauf describes how the character for Kidney, Shen 腎, means the organ in charge of kowtowing, Chen 臣, which depicts one acting with a noose around their neck, prostrate in complete surrender. We will be held prisoner, at least for a time during this life, to a sense of self, seemingly cut off from its source. The noose is woven of the infinite strands of the human chain, through our particular lineage with all of its gifts and challenges, all the way back to the first being.

The ninth phase of life challenges us to step up to a new potential and die to the old, so that we may reclaim our source. At the end of life, our physical Essence will wither to bones and teeth; so what constitutes the life that we have lived? Have we made use of what we were given? Have the threads of Heaven led us through our lessons and back to our source, or have they wrapped us up in contracted webs of fear and self concern? Similarly, in the ninth month of gestation, the baby must step up to the reality of its upcoming birth and all of its demands. Next month the womb will become a tomb, a fetus will die, and a baby will be born, with all the inner determination it will need to survive. It will also need to muster great strength, which the *Tao Te Ching (Book of the Way)* tells us is needed to master the self. As the fetus receives the energetics from the stone and engraves its own tombstone, the soul turns toward the challenges awaiting its future curriculum: *Am I going to accept the end of life in utero, and surrender to what Heaven decrees I must do to satisfy the criteria of this upcoming life? Am I willing to lose myself in order to find myself?* If the answer is no, we may have fetal death here. In some babies, however, the stimulation is so exciting, their eagerness may cause premature labor to ensue. Indecision may cause the baby to twist and turn until the cord wraps around its neck. In the usual case, though, the head bows to accept the figurative noose, and the head engages, capped by the sacred bone (sacrum) until it descends down the mysterious path of the birth canal, into the great unknown. This requires the greatest trust, given by the Kidneys.

The color given to the Kidneys is black, Xuan, whose character 玄 represents the dark mystery and depicts the silken threads woven from the source, tangible only by the Heart's ability to maneuver in the darkness where it can turn to a soundless, inner homing beacon. The gestating soul sees in the dark, a latent property that will be retained throughout its earthly life. One of our tasks in this life is to acquire the ability to inhabit our own darkness and let the light of Shen shine through so that we can find our way through whatever enigma life gives us.

Our brainstem's bias toward meeting the dictates of survival creates an inner pharmacy, whose neurochemicals will continue to magnetize us toward whatever negative, contracting issues we have yet to overcome in life, much of which is the residue from our own internalized parents. The Kidney's ability to consolidate can unite the polarities of chaos into wisdom, where we are given a new lease on life. Shifts in perception change the body's chemistry. Conversely, the contraction of unexamined fear can solidify our sense of self into compact hardness like bones and teeth, which will crumble and go into the ground while our spirit of aliveness, the soul, will have to recirculate again. The road to our destiny is tightly wrapped in the core of our DNA, where our deepest truth is known, tucked away in the basin of our lower Dan Tien, begging to be discovered, uncovered, and released.

While the soul has been gestating, hopefully the mother has been facing her own issues and clearing the way during the previous months of pregnancy. Her body and mind will need to be especially strong next month, so she is advised to cultivate conviction and certitude this month. She will need confidence as her very self, birther and mother. She will discover that she can do this thing, as she follows the long line of mothers who have been birthing babies back to the beginning. It's in her bones.

Completion in life implies that we have faced our fears and traced our steps back to the origin. Completion in utero means that the spatial cavities and energetic boundaries have been established; the hair is formed; uptake through the connecting thread, the umbilical cord is controlled; and nine Dan Tien chambers are established within the three Dan Tiens. The past, along with any issues of security and stability, has been programmed into the Essence of our constitution in the lower Dan Tien; future potential of how we utilize our Jing is encoded in the interactive energies of the middle Dan Tien; and the moment-to-moment expression of time carried out through life is expressed in the upper Dan Tien. Now is when we have access to eternity. The Jing–Shen axis is united through Yintang, which leans toward the prostrate posturing that actualizes the vision of the unitive third eye, and Baihui, which links to our cosmic home. These will be activated, although veiled, as the baby passes through the birth canal.

The Kidney meridian

The developing Kidney channel and its points represent the path that leads us to our destiny. Within it are three themes that correlate with the three compartments.

The points on the feet and legs represent stability and security. It takes courage and trust to be grounded in who we are and accept the force required to make the journey from our origin to our destination. Our Water energies must sustain us as we go out to find our fulfillment in life. When we lose our way or pick up inhibitions that hinder the force required to meet our destiny, the channel loops around the inner ankle so we can come back to meet any unresolved issues and reclaim our holy potential. Shen shines in the depths of our being; we reclaim ourselves, and journey onward.

As the channel emerges in the lower abdomen, our creative potential is called into life interactions, which may produce conflicts. The pelvis signifies a certain "gutter" of life that collects refuse to either be eliminated or recirculated. All that we can't handle goes into the Dai as a holding reservoir, or the Bao, where the vertical axis that organizes the fetus can reorganize our lives by vitalizing the Kidney potential. Since we reproduce what we are, as we change, so do our creations. Anything not resolved will be rebirthed. Heaven is "personified" as the Big Dipper, an interstellar deity that births us, governs our destiny, and calls us home. Chiseled into our belt is the first star of the Dipper, representing the junction between the Lower Jiao, which eliminates, and the middle, which nourishes. Here we can break through limitations and soothe distractions, so clear Qi can ascend with faith into the unknown, which is where we find our true purpose. At the Secret Gate, the heart can descend into the abyss to connect with the Kidneys and Chong Mai where we rise from the mysterious and dark depths of our own underbelly. This diaphragmatic transition place evokes our evolution from swimming creatures to land-dwelling bipeds; as belly water splashes against the land of the ribcage, so we ascend to the upper Spirit points where we can be fully awakened to the true virtue of Heaven within.

The energetics of the points on the chest represent the spirit of awakening to our true nature. The introspection represented by Water is brought to Fire in the intercostal spaces. As we step out onto the veranda of the ribcage, tranquilly protected from the harshness of life and the elements, and view how we've related to the experience of "me," we embrace a new view, where body, mind, and spirit come together as one. Our freedom of spirit may have been forfeited in order to fit in. But we can preserve our spirit until our inner certainty can be assured and integrated. If unresolved, our true spirit is buried until we dig out and revive the spirit that has lost its way and temporarily gone underground, depriving the soul of its rightful inheritance. And we rekindle the light, joy can return to pull us out of desperation and fear, reviving the Will. The spirits are lifted, and we are given wings enlivened with righteous elegance to reach the Upper Mansion, which holds the summation of our life's experiences, and where Jing and Shen are united. Inner conflicts resolved, no longer separate, creation responds directly to our pure impulses.

The Tao goes where one's head meets the path. The brain is a reflector that mirrors our journey. Te, the true virtue direct from the source, is a power given as one's bowed head is aligned over trusting feet, meeting in the heart. The sacred warp of Heaven is woven through the woof of every step; naturally and effortlessly embodying the wisdom of the Tao in the proper walk of life, humbly experienced as *I Am The Way*. Anything less is to squander the reason for being. This finality is being encoded in the Kidney channel this month.

As the uterus ascends toward its peak, the Great Gateway of Ren 14 Juque (Great Palace Gateway) is activated and the polar axis begins to shift, which will automatically begin to sever communication between the Heart and Kidneys so the baby can begin its descent. As Bao Mai loosens its connection with Bao Lou, mother and baby will seem to lose an inner sense of connection, as the Kidney no longer extends to reach up to the throat and tongue, but instead prepares to move toward the Yang of the Bladder to strategize its exit. The Heart also shifts its interest away from the lower crucible to communicate with the Small Intestine so it may prepare to transform Jing and Blood into milk, which will be needed to sustain this new life. It is thus advisable to avoid needling the Small Intestine channel until the tenth month.

As baby loses the communication with mother's Heart, the process of separation from the oceanic bliss of the cosmic womb begins, which will set it on its journey deeper into the underworld. Yet it is not lost; just as we know we all must die, the baby, guided by nature's urgings, knows it will be born. It doesn't lament; it moves on down to prepare for delivery. The Kidneys link us with our mysterious origin and the experience of unity with the macrocosm, which will now transfer to the microcosmic source energies, concentrated in the Yuan points, which can always be used to remind the being of its home when it loses its way. Now our baby must discover a new light, so its inward eye plunges into the depth of flesh as its head begins to orient toward the pure Yin at Ren 1 Huiyin (Meeting of Yin), until the lower light of the cervical opening is revealed. This journey leaves an imprint of how we must let go of previous bearings in order to follow the inner urgings of the Mysterious Mother down her passageway through the unknown, as Yin concentrates itself in the darkness until its own light begins to dazzle.

While the Sovereign Fire of the Heart no longer illuminates the Bao Lou, the baby, now capable of making its own noise, can call out underwater for another homing beacon. This process illustrates the necessity of using our own voice to find our way; only as we relinquish the voices of outer authorities can we speak our own autonomous truth. Meanwhile, the mother may feel as if her own Windows of Heaven are darkening and can, quite paradoxically, especially if the Kidneys are weak, lose her own voice. Here, we can use Liu Wei Di Huang Wan (Six Ingredient Pill with Rehmannia) along with the vine that passes through the night, Ye Jiao Teng (polygonum), to help restore her ability to speak, along with SJ 2 Yemen (Fluid Gate) and the heavenly prominence of Ren 22 Tiantu (Heavenly Rushing).

As far as the Kidneys are concerned, the opposite of fear is trust, especially of our inherent wisdom. Our greatest fear is that Heaven and Earth don't actually have our backs, that we are desperately alone in this world, and we may lose our way. Often this will come as a dark night when earthly things have lost their flavor. Our Taoist forebears have pointed out the worst consequence of fear is when we lose possession of ourselves. The Shen no longer have a place to rely on and thought becomes scattered. As the spirits take flight, we are no longer present in the Heart, and we lose the ability to know ourselves. The spirits are unable to express themselves and the vitality of Ming Men is shaken. As the Qi is disordered, there is separation.

The contraction of fear and all of its defensive postures prevent us from leaning into the winds of change that carry us along the path of our curriculum. It takes a lot of trust to break in one's Heart. The Zhi 志 spirit that belongs to the Kidneys steps in with courage and faith to plunge into what feels like chaos, daring to emerge into an uncertain future and reorganize a new potential. If we are rooted in the spirit of the Kidneys, we can accept Heaven's invitations through the trying circumstances of our own life as an opportunity to expand out of our contractions and thereby return to our cosmic origin.

Wind is said to be the source of a hundred diseases—one of the reasons is that it can blow us out of our comfort zone and invite us to change. You can feel Wind's urgings, but you can't grasp it. Like Wei Qi, Wind brings moods and sensations not necessarily of our own making. But like the pathogens Wind carries, they can share our DNA and disguise themselves as us. As Wind stirs, whether external or internal, it brings challenges to the previous order, and our response is paramount.

The Zhi (Will) is the power that focuses the Heart's intent into the material world. When it is in service to the first level, survival, we contract in fear. When the Will opens to the second level of relational dynamics, the soul expands into and is influenced by external people and circumstances; flowing with the winds of change may disrupt our present environment. Here we can see where outer circumstances have taken control of our lives. As our deepest mandate is to express our truth, we are invited to give up all outer authorities for inner autonomy. Just as mother and baby lose their connection during the ninth month, we may lose our sense of connection to the source, our creator, or that which gives authority to our lives. This may feel like despair, but if we don't resist or medicate, we can turn toward the goodness of Heaven within and find it can be trusted. As we turn to the goodness of Earth within, we find it can be trusted. And as we turn to the goodness of humanity, we find we can be trusted.

When the Will evolves to be uniquely itself in service to the all, the soul's porousness allows the winds of the universe to blow through, all the way down to the cellular level. From the Marrow outward, we respond to cosmic urgings with trust, which like Wei Qi, whose source is in the Kidneys, emerges on the surface. And we literally embody the wisdom and power, Te, of the pleroma, as the vessels of creation we were meant to be. Life steps in with its universal "yes" and the wings of the Heart ride the winds of change with great joy. When we have cultivated a state of being where we are in alignment with the ebb and flow of the elemental cycles of the natural world, we find our proper place in the natural order, where the cosmic, the psychic, and the physical are one.

In the ninth month, the mother *loosens her belt* and begins to wait for the right moment.

Proper positioning during the ninth month

In preparing for birth, we learn to descend into the unknown in order to find our way into life. In this phase of pregnancy the baby's head must descend and engage in the pelvic cavity as mom's chest opens to allow the downward release.

As the Shi (stone) is received, the fetus receives the Essence from the hundred joints. The most active of these joints is now the shoulder, a constitutional joint associated with the Yang Qiao and Wei Mai. LI 14 Binao (Upper Arm), LI 15 Jianyu

(Shoulder Bone), LI 16 Jugu (Great Bone), SI 10 Naoshu (Upper Arm Transporter), and SJ 15 Tianliao (Heavenly Crevice) can all help loosen the shoulders to remain active. The more Dampness the mother has been exposed to during the eighth and ninth month, the more the baby will move its shoulders to try to help dilate the mother's chest to rid of any Phlegm obstructing the way. This is one of the built-in mechanisms to open the Da Bao in order to release the Dai Mai to prepare for the descent of birth. This continuum allows you to treat mom's shoulders to address baby's shoulders, which then open mom's chest to help baby descend into its earthly life. This dynamic is also applicable any time we have difficulty clearing Dai Mai pathology. Sometimes we need to open the shoulders, chest, and upper back so the Da Bao can release what is held in the Dai Mai.

If the patient feels an achiness in the waist and low back, or urgent gripping of the abdomen with an energy rushing toward their Heart, it indicates the baby is having difficulty consolidating. E Jiao (ass-hide gelatin) can be used to help prevent early delivery. Don't needle or Moxa the Kidney channel and watch for too much Yin pathology like Dampness and Cold. During this time Ban Xia (pinellia) is the primary herb that can harmonize Rebellious Qi while clearing any residual Dampness, Cold, or Phlegm.

Malposition

Malpositioning can be due to a lack of Qi in the mother, which is addressed with Tu Si Zi (cuscuta), 24g. A rebellious baby is one who isn't able to engage properly. The major herb to address this is Dong Kui Zi (malvia), 24g, along with Niu Xi (acaranthus), 6g, and Da Huang (rhubarb root), 3g. If a baby isn't able to be oriented in the proper position, where Du 20 Baihui (Hundred Convergences) meets Ren 1 Huiyin (Meeting of Yin), it can cause disorientation between the Conception and Governing Meridians. It is important that the baby's head be pushed against the cervix and squeezed through the birth canal so that it swallows the "mud pill," which helps release the umbilical cord. During the birthing process, the mud pill then travels to the brain, which encourages the baby to take its first breath. If this process is bypassed, it may result in neurological symptoms or congenital conditions that disturb the Shen. It has been suggested that the plethora of caesarean sections correlate with the rise in attention deficits, obsessive, compulsive, and Autism spectrum disorders.

Breech presentations

When the baby reaches toward Ren 15 Jiuwei, a source point of Yin, the polar axis will tilt and shift toward Ren 1 Huiyin (Meeting of Yin). As the baby loses connection with the mother's Heart, it is meant to look for the light hidden in the deepest darkness. Supporting proper positioning will be crucial to help the baby find its way into the lower Yin, where it will be making its entrance into this dimension, or else it may continue to look upward, now a retrograde movement, for the prior light contained in its mother's Heart. The mother needs to open her chest and begin her process of release in order to help baby descend.

Insufficient or overabundant uterine fluid can contribute to the baby's failure to turn, as can uterine or placental abnormalities, maternal diabetes, and smoking. The baby's legs can be extended, flexed, or one of each. The skull may be felt in the subcostal area, which may become tender. During weeks 28 to 36, most babies spontaneously turn to a cephalic, or head down, presentation. If not, there is an increased risk of asphyxia and birth trauma.

In breech presentations the head fails to descend and remains pointed toward Heaven. In the way of Yin, of course, this is a no-no. Du 20 Baihui (Hundred Convergences) is connected to the spirit world and is meant to turn to meet Ren 1 Huiyin (Meeting of Yin) before it is birthed. A mother under considerable taxation won't be able to properly nurture the baby during the third trimester, which can impact the Wei Qi's ability to nourish the Liver sinews and cutaneous regions. In this case, we can nourish the Lung and Stomach Yin to promote Wei Qi in the Cou Li space, so it may turn to the earth.

Salt Moxa to Ren 8 Shenque (Spirit Palace Gateway) can help pivot the child toward the head-down position. UB 67 Zhiyin (Reaching Yin) is the final Yang on the Yang Bladder channel. Zhi Yin is Yin's extreme, where we find the unique depth of our inner nature. At Yin's utmost, the darkness moves until it ignites an internal pathway that illuminates our way from within. Acupuncture to UB 67 Zhiyin from 32 to 36 weeks along with daily self-administered moxibustion agitates the fetus to increase the likelihood of repositioning.

MOTHERS' GUIDELINES FOR THE NINTH MONTH
Nutrition

- Eat small amounts of moist and nutritious foods.

- Make sure there is enough bulk and roughage in the diet to move your bowels.
- Adding more fat to your diet is good for your baby's developing nervous system.
- If you like organ meat, pig's kidneys are recommended this month.
- Drink a little wine to help invigorate the Blood.
- Make sure you drink plenty of fluids.
- Supplement your diet with added magnesium and vitamin D.

Lifestyle and exercises

- Wear loose clothing.
- Make sure there is no restriction around your waist.
- Speak up about what's important to you in birthing this baby.
- Make sure you are getting plenty of rest.
- Keep exercising your perineal and levator ani muscles. When you sit, press the bone behind your big toe to the floor while simultaneously lifting your pelvic floor.
- Do some pelvic rotations to strengthen and open your pelvis.
- Focus on your feet and encourage your baby to follow a downward movement, directing his or her head toward the ground.
- Rotate your torso in horizontal circles to open your chest.
- Lift and lower your arms to your sides to exercise your shoulder muscles.
- Circle your shoulders and shoulder girdle. Notice any resistant or stuck places, and stay with them until they open up.
- Exercise your voice by humming to yourself.
- Return your inner dialog to yourself.
- When you experience preparatory contractions, practice breathing into the discomfort with short and rapid breaths.

Self-inquiry exercises

- This month is about acceptance and making peace with the last nine months. Is there anything you need to forgive and relinquish?
- How do you feel about your upcoming birthing process?

- In what ways can you let go of your baby as he or she prepares for the birthing process?
- Name any fears you have—not only about the upcoming labor, but any other seemingly unrelated insecurities that may be creeping up.
- In what ways do you trust yourself?
- In what ways do you distrust yourself?
- Are there any areas in your life where you feel you are lacking security and stability?
- Do you feel resistance to any of the upcoming changes required of you?
- How can you accept any conflicting energies without trying to resolve them and find a place of peace and grace?

CHAPTER 16

Urinary Bladder: Lunar Month Ten

Weeks 36–40

Days 253–280

> Hundun awaits in the ancient basin of chaos, where her giant son
> Pangu stirs the cosmic egg into separation.
> The River Qing, laden with jade, emerges from Kunlun mountain.
> There is a twinge; something new; surrender is the only option.
> The first mother appears, attended by
> the quilin, turtle, phoenix and dragon.
> At the lower Yin, Nuwa opens the gate
> and the milky way ascends to Heaven.

Birthing is not just an event but a process. It is a microcosmic reflection of the macrocosmic arising where eons ago, the eight winds, previously at rest, began to stir, producing a current through which the Tao was quickened into being. Swirling gasses formed into star seeds, which eventually burst into whole galaxies. Their collision gave rise to planetary orbs, through which all the elements necessary for life emerged. The creation of the universe happens in every cell, every moment. The cosmic body is our body, and it will continue to evolve. Until I have met everything within myself, until *my* story becomes *the* story, it's not finished.

The conclusion of our birthing story begins as labor approaches, but continues beyond the expulsion of the baby. The gestating woman and fetus must "die" to life in utero as they plunge into a deep surrender to the Mysterious Mother who has never left them, and never will, for she has always given birth to all things. Deep in our cells, we can tap into our indwelling link to the original mother. The divine awakens capacities that only she can fulfill. The spiritual longing for life is a most terrible agony, challenging us in ways that nothing else can, as the separate self has no power to fulfill it on its own. We do not regenerate our own souls. We tend only to the death of the old, trusting there will be a new arising. And like the character Ling 靈, the priestesses dance themselves into the state from whence our souls all vibrated into existence, and usher the unborn into being.

Every time a new consciousness is being birthed, the center of our earthly being first destabilizes, so something new can erupt. This can be likened to Pangu trying to hold up the pillars of the sky as the old world crumbles, leaving gaping holes in Heaven. Birthing new realms unsettles the previous order. The fabric of our being is torn apart; the sky of our mental realm can no longer stay together. What a gloriously courageous process. The birthing of the new always requires relinquishing the old.

In order to gain access, we can inquire within: Do we dare enter into this brave and uncharted new land? While our fiercest selves are being called forth, what is actually needed? Probably not medication and intervention, but rather, relinquishing control of our inner orbit through a deeper surrender that turns our insides out. Awakening through the birthing process is painful and messy. As our narratives that keep Heaven and Earth in their place are challenged, we may become disoriented. There's nothing to do but lean into the discomfort and call upon the Mother. The self-made costume unravels and the funeral banner flies away. There's nothing left of the old self. So don the winged garment of the Tao and give birth to the Mother, incarnate love.

Remember, birthing is a descent, not an ascent. The human crown, with the potential for the highest good, responds to gravity and follows the low places, like Water. And here we are schooled by the divine composer to move into the pain, where we find deeper and more profound transformative qualities, and greater openings to the divinity found in the depths. The mother must learn to honor this new stirring within herself, uncomfortable as it may be, by turning toward it. She gives herself to the same love that is the longing for life itself, disguised as the pain of contraction. Pain doesn't always mean something's wrong. Just as often it indicates the emergence of something new or unmet.

As we enter this last month, the five fully formed Zang, six Fu, and umbilicus are connected. Fetal education is complete, and the baby has been acted upon with favorable Essences of Heaven and Earth. The Qi of Heaven and Earth settles into the lower Dan Tien where they refine the Essences in order to finalize a Ren Shen, a full and spirited human being. Completion of the "articulations and relays" are part of this process, which refers to the way the baby has been programmed to perceive and move in the world and through which it will grasp its new reality.

The Bao has woven the threads of the universe into material form; the wrapping is now complete. The vertical threads of the warp will continue to connect to Heaven, while the horizontal woof secures to the Earth, veiling it with a perceptual experience of time and space through which Shen will live out this particular life. The soul will now be unfastened from the cosmic loom.

Expelling this baby, like any other death/rebirth, requires a tremendous amount of Qi. This month is one of rest and expectant waiting, for *the lord and master resides in non-action.* Consider it practice for Wu Wei 無 or "non-doing," a state of being in which actions are effortlessly aligned with the ebb and flow of the elemental cycles of the natural world. Non-action moves us into an internal state where the light rotates according to its own law around the central channel where we are directly plugged into the source. When we free up our contract with what binds us in life (which we've been doing throughout), we can enter a state of pure spontaneity. Inner cultivation calms the body and mind, allowing the sage to align with heavenly dynamism and act like Water—supple and non-striving, a liquid symmetry that follows the natural order. Those who develop these principles become authentic—real, straight from the source, not a copy of anything or anyone else. Like an uncarved block, they embrace simplicity and *do not interfere with the nature of things*. In awake ease, wisdom appears in the moment perfectly appropriate to whatever situation arises. This is the natural state, which has its own power, and its own timing.

Rest and waiting augment the Yuan Jing until it has the force required to transform the fetus into a baby and release it from its maternal envelope into the world. Qi Hua is the energy of transformation that carries the power to make the mundane celestial, and it is governed by the Urinary Bladder, which regulates the pressure of holding and releasing, transforms Qi, and stores liquids.

The Urinary Bladder, Pang Guang, was originally written as 旁光, ferry light, referring to the bladder's function of ushering prenatal Essence up the spine to ignite the enlightened glow of Shen in the upper Sea of Marrow. When, through disciplined tantric practices, retained Essences are not expelled outside the body, the resulting hormonal changes produce all kinds of favorable transformative effects. On "Safeguarding Prenatal Energy," the *Nei Jing* speaks of self-realized (male) masters controlling the quintessential forces of the universe by holding, concealing, storing away, and through extraordinary internal focus congealing their Essence in the lower Dan Tien. Likewise, when a woman congeals the universe into a fetus and retains it in the lower Dan Tien for three-quarters of a year, it will incite great changes in the middle and upper Dan Tien as well. When Leg Tai Yang, magnificent like the sun, has ripened it thoroughly, it will harness all of the Yang power required to expel it, while Arm Tai Yang Small Intestine carries the Essence to the breasts.

It is decreed that the divine process of accouchement is designed to change the life of its recipient, as her Heart-Mind is opened to become more receptive to the frequency of a future reality. As the mother houses this child of tomorrow, she is meant to undergo her own transformation. Her old ideas and beliefs are often challenged as she is crafted into an expanded version of herself, capable of responding to a yet unrealized potential. The one who gives birth is not the same one through whom conception occurred. She no longer dwells in the land of yesterday. Over the last nine months she's been made aware of and relinquished certain limitations and blocks within herself. As she has received herself fully, she no longer perceives herself as the isolated entity she had taken herself to be. She is a unique microcosm of the macrocosm, ready for creation to use her as its vehicle through which it can mold future generations.

Free of limiting beliefs, she can now become aware of the purity of her own consciousness, prior to any body or mind functioning. This consciousness is uniquely hers and yet not separate from anything. Shen, pure consciousness, perceives all sensations, thoughts, and emotions, without judgment. It's only afterwards that the mind steps in to offer its opinions, like *This hurts too much. I can't do it.* When she is rooted in spirit, Ben Shen, she has the power to be fully present with whatever is happening and can lean fully into the heightened sensations of the birthing process. Without resistance, the unobstructed opening of the cervix can send waves of intensity through her system that the mind can interpret as either extremely painful or fiercely orgasmic. If she is not utilizing epidural or opioid pain medication, her system will be flooded with high levels of endogenous endorphins, producing euphoric states of consciousness.

Today hospital births and birthing centers have become the norm, Yet, as we gain understanding of the birthing process dynamics, we can see why it is not a necessity to have medical professionals present during the baby's sacred welcome into the world. Just because medical intervention is available doesn't mean we all should utilize it all the time. This is an exciting time, but doesn't need to be fearful, which preparing for emergencies tends to be. Many women without complicated pregnancies are choosing to have free births, where they and their partner are in control over the setting, usually at home, perhaps with a doula to provide birthing support. Access to trained maternity care providers should be available to provide medical management plans as needed.

Birthing isn't something that can be learned. It is a knowing deep inside, held within the wisdom of the womb. A long line of mothers down the maternal line have been birthing babies, all the way back to the first mother. In kind, this mother has learned to move into, rather than away from, the wisdom of her body's sensations. Her only job is to breathe, trust, and surrender. As she opens her heart to the experience, the rest of her body can follow. She softens. There is no separation. She, the baby, and the Tao are One, and are meant to flow through this process like Water. The same force that's been growing this baby has the power to expel it. The Valley Spirit, the Mysterious Feminine, when called upon, offers up Yang Qi with a geyser-like force so she won't have to push the baby through this inter-dimensional strait alone.

As she lets go into the inevitable, her baby must, too. In the oceanic bliss of the perinatal matrix, the mother has been providing the Essence of all of the baby's survival functions as it has grown from a mere inkling into a human child, now encroaching on the mother's sternum where it can't rise any higher. Soon, the baby will have to switch its reliance to the Qi of its own Dan Tien in order to breathe, eat, and keep itself warm. The only world it has known is closing in on it. Cramped and confined, it has turned toward the lower Yin. Cut off from the mother's Heart, it now begins to emit chemicals of distress that communicate with the mother's endocrine system to induce hormonal changes that will trigger oxytocin production and initiate labor, causing the palace of the baby to squeeze its walls in even further, causing it to enter the Mysterious Pass, an event horizon between realities. Here it will be expelled into the world, ready to live out its destiny.

The moment the star seeds of the cosmos were captured by the embrace of Yin and Yang, it was portended through the precise alignment of the heavenly bodies just when, where, and how the macrocosm would emerge as this new human being. That time has come. But first, the emerging baby must pass through one more portal. Its life force will be withdrawn, and it will be separated from all it has known. It will be compressed into more darkness. Recall *The Secret of the Golden Flower*'s instruction: *When the dark is at rest the light begins to move.* Each contraction will interrupt the supply of blood and oxygen. Increasing in intensity, all she can do is let the process take her over.

In the vast space between the strands of her DNA, she knows how to do this for this is the natural law. She has all of creation behind her. Seemingly against all hope, she continues on toward this new light. Her crown knocks upon the birth gate. Her head, round like Heaven, will squeeze through the cervix, followed by her body, square like earth. Against striking odds, a human being will come to be.

> If you want to be born, you first must die.
> If you want to be given everything, give everything up.
>
> —*Tao Te Ching (Book of the Way), Chapter 22*

Saint John of the Cross, in his essay, "The Ascent of Mount Carmel," states something similar to Lao Tzu. In various stanzas, he recapitulates that to come to the possession of something new, or what you have not, you must go by a way that you know not. If, however, you turn toward any particular desire, you cease to "cast yourself upon the all." In all new birthing endeavors, we must travel a path that we know not, even if we have done this before. Each time we enter the void, it's always brand spanking new.

MOTHERS' GUIDELINES FOR THE TENTH MONTH
The mother's tasks will be few this month, as she has already been preparing for this for the previous nine months. As labor approaches, however, she is advised to:

- Consume very little or no sugar.
- Abstain from alcohol.
- Practice rapid and shallow breathing, which activates the Wei Qi.

There will likely be ambivalent feelings about the upcoming delivery. While there will be a knowing that it's okay to trust this process, there will also likely be some doubts and misgivings.

Self-inquiry exercises

- What part of you wants to believe you aren't capable of this?
- What do you need to be ready to release this message?
- What part of you knows that you can do this?
- What does that part need for support?

Remember always to lean into the discomfort and breathe. You have everything you need within you.

- Where are any fears holding you back from creating the environment you and your baby deserve?
- What do you need in order to replace fear with trust?
- How can you make this birthing process sacred?

Preparing for labor

During the delivery process, Yang Qi will need to be summoned, for which Du Zhong (eucommia) may be prescribed or added to applicable herbal formulas this month. The mother would do well to avoid cold weather, drinking alcohol, eating cold foods, or overdoing any activities that might exhaust her Yang Qi.

Just like a corpse is prepared for its funeral and burial, the fetus prepares for its prenatal death, where it will release the casing of its mother in order to step up to accept its own life as a new heavenly being. The baby's hormones initiate labor, which the mother's hypothalamus perceives and responds to by sending chemical messages to the posterior pituitary gland to release oxytocin, to which the uterus, in turn, responds by squeezing down and opening up the birth gate. Oxytocin causes uterine contractions and milk ejection, and also triggers prolactin secretion, which is responsible for milk production. Painful contractions can be eased with auricular points, especially Shenmen and Uterus as well as needling any other red or inflamed points on the ear.

During the first phase of labor, as the mother's body begins to let go of the fetus, her cervix will first thin and stretch out through a process called effacement. It subsequently and sometimes concurrently dilates from a closed state to a diameter of approximately 10 centimeters in order to accommodate the passage of the baby. Walking around, sitting and moving on an exercise ball, rotating or swaying the hips can help open the pelvic girdle to assist with cervical dilation.

While early in pregnancy, Hua Tai (slippery fetus) is considered a risk for loss; a slippery fetus can now ease its way through the birth canal like a fish. Chuan Bei Mu (frittelaria), Dang Kui Zi (malvia), Hua Shi (talcum), and Niu Xi (acyranthes) all help to make the fetus slippery. Dong Kui Zi (malvia) is the main herb to bring things to completion. Associated with Water, it ends the winter cycle before Wood initiates birth. Adding Che Qian Cao (plantain) and Niu Xi (acyranthes) can help speed up delivery and move downward. Bai Shao Tang (White Peony Root Decoction) consists of Bai Shao (white peony), Dang Gui (angelica), Chuan Xiong (cnidium), Bai Zhu (atractylodes), and Huang Qin (skullcap root), all in equal amounts. Similar to Sang Shen Fang (Ripen the Baby Formula), which we discussed during the eighth month, Dan Shen Gao (salvia paste) incorporates 24g of Dan Shen (salvia), 9g of both Dang Gui and Chuan Xiong, and Sichuan pepper if they need more Yang, or Ma Zi Ren (hemp seed) or Hai Zhi Ma (black sesame seeds) if they need more Yin.

Sun Si Miao also recommended powdering 24g of Che Qian Zi (plantago seeds) with E Jiao (ass-hide gelatin) and Hua Shi (talcum), and taking one teaspoon twice per day to dilate the cervix and promote discharge of the baby. He also recommended kissing, sexual stimulation, and orgasm, which encourages the release of oxytocin from the pituitary gland to initiate or increase uterine contractions.

The *Bei Ji Qian Jin Yao Fang* (*Essential Prescriptions worth a Thousand in Gold for Every Emergency*) addressed birthing difficulties that delayed labor with relatively simple herbal formulas like:

- Chi Xiao Dou (phaseolus seed) and E Jiao (ass-hide gelatin).
- Huai Zi (sophorica japonica) and Pu Huang (typhae pollen).
- Sheng Di Huang (rehmannia) and Sheng Jiang (ginger).

In more severe delays, as when labor extended into days, charred rat's head, axle grease, and straw soiled from the privy were given, as well as having her husband blow in her mouth 14 times to dislodge the baby. While we might scoff at such nonsense, it isn't all that different from women taking probiotics, going into high altitudes, or drinking castor oil to bring on labor.

While the climate of the times has changed, it has always been clear that birthing exposes the mother and baby to major risks and potential loss of life. Yet when mother and baby have been cared for throughout pregnancy, there are far fewer risks than in one with no prenatal care. It also decreases the likelihood of birth trauma, which lodges in the Chong Mai, manifesting as poor instincts, a negative outlook on life, an inability to connect with one's body, and using external relationships to compensate for the most important one—with oneself.

The birthing process

You are being invited into the womb space where all true transformations occur. These invitations will continue throughout your life, where you will be urged to release your defenses to the inevitable pain of living life fully enough to become your true self. Release your hold as you enter the birth realm so you may merge with the Mysterious Mother, who unhooks you from your previous moorings, so you may expand beyond your present boundaries. You may now exit the palace.

The baby is engaged in position when the widest part of its head has entered the pelvis. During the second stage of labor, the baby moves through the vaginal canal. In the easiest and most common cephalic presentation, the rear of baby's head is positioned down and toward the front, its chin is tucked into its chest, and it faces the mother's back. Its spine is longitudinal and its arms and legs are folded in toward the center of its chest. Any other delivery presentation may stall progression through the pelvis and the obstetrician may elect surgical delivery. This will, of course, hinder the necessary passage through the birth canal. The baby's head descends further through the pelvis as the cervix dilates, and its head usually turns while one shoulder is down and the other up. The head then extends back and rotates.

The top part of the uterus actively contracts downward, while the lower portion remains passive. When the head appears through the vaginal opening, it is called crowning. The mother pushes during active contractions, during which time the baby's head may elongate. The head turns as it emerges, then the shoulders spiral out one after the other, followed by the rest of the body. Finally, in the third stage, the placenta will be expelled.

During the birthing process, ancient obstetricians used to carry flying squirrel pelts or the heads of certain birds in order to hasten delivery from the pre-heavenly dimension into the post-heavenly dimension. The bed was positioned according to the most auspicious celestial and terrestrial alignments to facilitate a rapid exit. They would call to the baby, "Fai fai chu lai," meaning "Quickly, quickly, come out," to summon a rapid exit. Birthing is a traumatic event, both physically and psychologically. It's meant to be. Like any shamanic journey, it takes one to the realm between worlds. For the baby it will mean loss of buoyancy, the exposure to the harshness of light, and severing its life support. For the mother, it may trigger her own birth trauma, which is held in the Chong Mai. If she hasn't used this time to discover, uncover, and release her own blockages, she will most certainly encounter them now.

Acupuncture isn't meant to "induce" labor; the baby is. Acupuncture is used to facilitate a natural process that has its own divine timing. When we are called upon to hasten a rapid and smooth labor, certain treatment considerations can guide us to address any deficient or stuck energies that may delay the onset or progression of labor. Yet we don't want parturition to be delayed either, as the Blood of an overdue pregnancy can become stagnant and toxic, so we may need to nudge things along.

Lv 3 Taichong (Great Surge) can help get the Qi moving, and LI 4 Hegu (Joining Valley) stimulates the uterus and addresses shoulder presentations. St 36 Zusanli (Leg Three Miles) moves the bowels and activates the Qi, Sp 6 Sanyinjiao (Three Yin Intersection) encourages uterine contractions and irritates the baby, SJ 5 Waiguan (Outer Pass) can be used to release the exterior, and GB 21 Jianjing (Shoulder Well) can transform turbidity to help dislodge the mucous plug, relax the sinews, and descend the Qi. Duyin, under the second toe, can also stimulate contractions and initiate labor. UB 60 Kunlun (Kunlan Mountains), a point that is used during the dying process to call the spirit home, also facilitates prenatal death and birth.

Once contractions begin, the mother will likely be uncomfortable staying in one position for very long, so don't expect to treat her in a relaxed and horizontal position. In China and most other Indigenous cultures, birthing is done in a squatting position, not lying down. Labor treatments are active, dynamic, and moving. Sometimes you will put in one or two needles and she will need to shift positions, or a change will occur requiring you to withdraw them and recheck the pulses to see how labor is progressing. Other applicable treatment principles depend upon specific diagnostic factors. Some questions you might ask include:

- Is the Lung Qi descending to the Lower Jiao? If the right Guan pulse is wiry and the Lungs are uncommunicative with the Kidney, encourage deep diaphragmatic breathing. Then stimulate Lu 7 Lieque (Broken Sequence), the opening point of the Conception Vessel, to descend the Lung Qi.
- Is there intense back labor? Does the pulse feel stuck on the superficial level? SI 3 Houxi (Back Stream) opens up the Governing Vessel. You may pair with UB 62 Shenmai (Extending Vessel) or the opening point of any other applicable extraordinary vessel. Reducing Du 14 Dazhui (Great Vertebra) may help open the neck, clear Heat, and help the Wei Qi descend down the back. UB 40 Weizhong (Supporting Middle) and UB 57 Chengshan (Mountain Support) can be used to open the tailbone, and UB 31 Shangliao (Upper Crevice) and UB 32 Ciliao (Second Crevice) can facilitate release.
- Is there a stall causing intense waist pain? It may help to open and release the Dai Mai. Reduce GB 41 Zulinqi (Foot Governor of Tears), and massage, Moxa, or lightly needle GB 26 Daimai (Girdle Vessel), GB 27 Wushu (Five Pivots), or GB 28 Weidao (Linking Path).

Yang Qi is mustered up to open the portal between worlds. Moxabustion to the Yang channel's Jing Well points, which open the orifices and shift states of consciousness, can assist and address any unforeseen stalls, but the general rule is not to use them until the mother feels the contractions throughout the entire Dai Mai, including the back. Given in order of the reverse Sheng cycle, we commence with Water and end with Wood.

UB 67 Zhiyin (Reaching Yin) can ground the baby by helping to position its Du 20 Baihui (Hundred Convergences) at the mother's Ren 1 Huiyin (Meeting of Yin). When the Dai Mai experiences labor pains, use LI 1 Shangyang (Metal

Yang). The Large Intestine impacts how the palace of the child will pulse open its gate, and just as LI 1 Shangyang opens the canal of the throat, it is mirrored by opening the birth canal. Metal descends the Qi, inducing the baby to push against the cervix. As the baby knocks at its door, we shift to St 45 Lidui (Sick Mouth), which encourages the mouth of the uterus, the cervix, to properly position itself into a dilated position. SI 1 Shaoze (Lesser Marsh) helps the baby to separate from its old environment, and also promotes lactation. SJ 1 Guanchong (Rushing Pass) helps the abdominal energies rise to the chest to facilitate the expulsion of the baby, especially when the mother is ambivalent or nervous, which can generate Wind Phlegm and prevent oxytocin release. When retrograde afterbirth retreats inward and doesn't let go, GB 44 Zuqiaoyin (Yin Portals of the Foot) can help expel the placenta and prevent postpartum depression. If residual lochia is not discharged, it can create Dampness and Cold in the uterus, which can lead to postpartum stagnation and depression.

Use these interventions as necessary; you will never need all of them. In sync with the mother's ability to release, the baby exits the palace. The baby has crossed the sovereign threshold and has made it to the promised land. The spirit of the universe has once again become human. A year old already, the baby lets out a cry of triumph.

As the baby emerges, skin-to-skin contact should be facilitated on the mother's bare chest. The baby will often root to begin feeding on the breast, and its focus will often magnetize to mom's eyes. This is an important bonding time. As baby's mouth and eyes are engaged, its Conception Meridian and mirror neurons are being established, which will internalize its external environment into its new inner landscape. Nursing will facilitate uterine contractions and help expel the placenta. To enhance the baby's Wei Qi, it is encouraged to keep the umbilical cord intact for a few minutes after birth, until the baby is able to breathe on its own and the cord stops pulsating. Not only does the placenta continue to deliver more blood and immunologic cells while the baby is being exposed to its new environment, if the cord is cut before the first breath ignites the fire of San Jiao, the baby can go into an instinctual panic because its independent energy production hasn't taken over yet. Let's take it as slow and easy as we can. We have made it all the way from the void through the birth gate.

Postpartum

Sun Si Miao, in the *Bei Ji Qian Jin Yao Fang*, considered childbirth, like menstrual blood, to be spiritually polluting. The ground on which a woman labored was to be covered in grass to keep the turbid birthing blood off the ground, which might offend the spirits. The mother wasn't allowed to look at the baby or the afterbirth, or to know the baby's gender, in case it might disappoint her. Severe restrictions prohibited her from engaging in life, and she was strictly forbidden from being exposed to people who might be depressed or in mourning. While we might agree that she should be protected and allowed to rest, these misogynistic taboos might have been an early attempt to allay postpartum depression.

A miracle has just manifested, but the process is far from over. In some ways it has just begun, and it is a very vulnerable time for the mother. The macrocosm has become a microcosm and the birth gate begins to close. She has been turned inside out, emptied of her baby, her hormones plunge, and from this new state, her neurotransmitters will be reset. Moods are often depressed when one's previous reality is withdrawn, when one has gone to the underworld and back, where the heavenly dimensions have opened the mother up to create life and her entire being has just been transformed. She has seen, first hand, that parts of her were figments of her own imagination, and she is experiencing withdrawal from her own internal chemical pharmacy of her previous reality. There is simply no returning to the way things used to be, nor should we expect elevated moods. Before we are too quick to pathologize and medicate what's going on, let's first imagine being held in this low state, with the assurance that this is natural, as we wait for a new order to establish itself. The moon goes dark before it waxes again. Our mother has been reborn and is being rewired.

Oxytocin, a peptide hormone that acts as a neurotransmitter, floods her system, stimulating milk production and release, contracting the uterus, and promoting bonding. In some, this produces relaxation and joy, the emotion of the Heart. In others, shifting the energy to the Heart can intensify any related deficiency or excess. Check the Heart pulse to see if it's bound or deficient, and assess if the Liver Blood and Qi are able to keep up with the hormones that need to be metabolized. Further, she's likely to be exhausted. Regardless of how intensely this baby is wanted, not everyone is elated to fully embrace the responsibility for another human being for the next couple of decades, and may be overwhelmed, consciously or subconsciously, by its enormity.

So let's let her be, as we supplement what's weak, build the Blood, fortify the Spleen, nourish the Heart and spirit, address obstructions in the Da Bao, and practice our craft. We are still supporting the creation of a new human being. The mother is to be nourished, held, and heard. Any little shocks around this time can destabilize her. Ideally, she will be supported by partners, parents, friends, or siblings to help out with the baby and care for her while she is allowed to rest. She should sleep propped up with pillows and have her legs elevated so everything can return back to the Dai for a few days. Over the next 100 days or so she has a lot to integrate.

Create your own rituals for your patients during their treatments. All acupuncture can be ritualistic if performed in the right spirit. Let them share their birth process with you. The ancient ceremony of "closing the bones" honors the immense opening the mother has just been through, part of which includes swaddling her like a chrysalis in warm wraps, and calling her spirit back. This will help create closure, and seal any leaking Qi, especially around the hips and pelvis, the Doorways to Earth, as she returns to the Sheng cycle to support her new baby.

You can massage and warm doorways to Earth points, like UB 40 Weizhong (Supporting Middle), Ki 11 Henggu (Pubic Bone), GB 30 Huantiao (Jumping Round), Lv 12 Jimai (Swift Pulse), St 30 Qichong (Surging Qi), Sp 12 Chongmen (Rushing Gate), Ren 1 Huiyin (Meeting of Yin), Ren 4 Guanyuan (Origin Pass), Du 1 Pomen (Long Strong), and Du 4 Mingmen (Gate of Destiny), which have particular resonance to the lower orifices, perhaps with essential oils. This can prevent the development of latent pathology. You may also balance with Windows of Heaven points, choosing the most appropriate points from Du 16 Fengfu (Wind Mansion), UB 10 Tianzhu (Celestial Pillar), SI 16 Tianchuang (Heavenly Window), SI 17 Tianrong (Celestial Appearance), SJ 16 Tianyou (Window of Heaven), LI 18 Futu (Support the Prominence), St 9 Renying (Person's Welcome), Lu 3 Tianfu (Heavenly Residence), Pc 1 Tianchi (Heavenly Pool), and Ren 22 Tiantu (Heavenly Rushing), which resonate with the upper orifices, to reestablish harmony with the mind.

Her diet is to include warm, nourishing, and easy-to-digest foods that build back the Qi and Blood. Food should be served around room temperature—not too hot or cold—and should include lots of fruit and vegetables. Chinese black chicken soup (from black-boned or silky chickens) is the classic postpartum recipe, which, in addition to the marrow-rich bone broth that supplements the

Yuan level, is also mineral and antioxidant-rich. Make sure she is well hydrated. If she hasn't been supplementing with omega-3 fatty acids, folic acid, Vitamins B and D, they all can help, as can dark chocolate, almonds, and Hu Lu Ba (fenugreek seeds).

Postpartum herbal support focuses on supplementing the Qi and Blood, as the Zang organs are in a vacuous condition and more vulnerable to Wind invasion. She is not to expose herself to the elements or to have sex. Unless specific issues requiring draining treatments are required, they are otherwise to be avoided. Tonifying medicinals are not to be consumed until seven days postpartum. Over the next 100 days, the baby's Ren Mai will be established, where it will be imprinted with all of its maternal surroundings. Meanwhile, mom is in a state of recovery. Not only will her Qi and Blood need to be replenished, but her open Heart will simultaneously be imprinted with a new reality, supplied by the pure love and oneness of her baby's consciousness, yet untainted by earthly illusions.

After birth, meaty soups and brews are often prepared with Qi and Blood-tonifying herbs like Huang Qi (astragalus) and Dang Gui (angelica). Other postpartum formulas include:

- Si Shun Li Zhong Wan (Four Arrangements to Regulate the Middle Pill): Gan Cao (licorice), Ren Shen (ginseng), Bai Zhu (atractylodes), Gan Jiang (ginger).
- Tao Ren Jian (Peach Pit Decoction): Tao Ren (peach kernel) powdered and added to high-grade liquor; simmer for 24 hours. Take with partner.
- Shi Hu Di Huang Jian (Dendrobian and Rehmannia Decoction): Shi Hu (dendrobium), Sheng Di Huang Zhi (rehmannia juice), Tao Ren (peach kernel), Gui Xin (cinnamomum cassia), Gan Cao (licorice), Da Huang (rhubarb root), Zi Wan (asteris), Mai Men Dong (ophiopogon), Fu Ling (poria), and Chun Jiu (pure grain spirit).

Postpartum complications
Retained placenta
The Metal Jing Well point of the Gallbladder, GB 44 Zuqiayin (Yin Portals of the Foot), has the added function of helping to release retained placenta from the uterus:

- Niu Xi (achyranthes root), Qi Mai (dianthus), Hua Shi (talcum), Dang Gui (angelica), Tong Cao (tetrapanax), and Dong Kui Zi (malvia).
- Fu Xiao Mai (tritici fructus) and Chi Xiao Dou (phaseolus seed).
- Niu Xi (achyranthes root) and Dong Kui Zi (malvia).
- Ban Xia (pinellia) and Bai Lian (ampelopsis japonica).

Postpartum bleeding

While the cause will need to be ascertained (Heat, stasis, Qi deficiency), Sp 10 Xuehai (Sea of Blood) addresses many Blood disorders. The following herbs are almost always included in the formulas that address the underlying pattern:

- E Jiao (ass-hide gelatin) and Pu Huang (typhae pollen).

Lactation

The bioactive proteins in breast milk enhance gut and brain health and immune development. The nursing process also reduces the rates of cardio and vascular issues in the mother, as well as the propensity for cancers of the breast.

Throughout the second and third trimesters, estrogen, progesterone, and prolactin have been preparing the mammary glands for milk production. After delivery, as estrogen and progesterone drop, prolactin takes over. Then oxytocin, a hormone that acts as a neurotransmitter in response to feelings of trust, intimacy, and skin-to-skin touch, stimulates the movement of the uterus and breasts and pushes milk out of the ducts. These Heart-based movements belong to the Small Intestine. The goddess knows herself through connection, and a woman's power center is in her Heart. As her energy shifts from the lower Dan Tien and "the Milky Way ascends," digestive energies will be transferred via the Small Intestine to the middle Dan Tien where her Heart energies will infuse the breast milk with the true nutrition of love. Low milk production is associated with Qi and especially Blood deficiency. If oxytocin release is inhibited, SI 1 Shaoze (Lesser Marsh) can redirect the inner light to open the flow of milk, as can these herbal approaches:

- Small doses of Mai Ya (barley sprout) (large doses inhibit lactation).
- Shi Zhong Ru (stalactite), Bai Shi Zhi (kaolin), Tong Cao (tetrapanax), Jie Geng (platycodon), Xiao Shi (niter, mineral form of potassium nitrate).
- Shi Gao (gypsum).

- Mai Men Dong (ophiopogon), Shi Zhong Ru (stalactite), Tong Cao (tetra-panax), Li Shi (fibrous gypsum).

Remain adrift on the ocean of birth and death
connected to the dark source
where there is no need to conform;
honor your uniqueness
as you alone
drink from the Great Mother's breasts.

—*Adapted from Chapter 20 of Tao Te Ching (Book of the Way)*

Conclusion

The cosmic body has given itself fully for this soul's incarnation, as it does every time. The hope of something unseen has shaped itself in the womb of humanity, wrapped itself into flesh, and become a someone, with the pure potential of the Tao at its disposal to reach its own authentic destiny, which is ultimately our collective destiny.

This child will play and dance, have hopes and dreams, and fall in love. Its Qi and Blood will be patterned by convention, and it will close down parts of its soul to develop an ego. It will feel small and scared, will stumble through heartbreak, and lose its way. Its parents will inevitably cast a net of hopes and expectations upon it, and try to condition it according to their highest view, which is not its own. But if it dares to meet itself fully as its mother has, if it will be brave enough to descend through its own darkness, its inviolable Shen will shine through the Jing, and it will discover a new source of light that can illuminate the Way for all that come behind.

Go far, little soul, give yourself fully to this beautiful earthly life; taste its bounties and respect the natural order, and above all else, become who you are. Teach your parents well and remind them of who they are. Keep your feet on the ground, your head in the stars, and challenge your Heart to reach beyond its limitations until the only thing left to do is to sing and dance the song of creation. Then you will see it all as a reflection of Yourself. You are a part of a larger story. You are the sun; you are the moon. The whole universe is within you. Use it as you will; the infinite source will never run dry. You were born for this.

Epilogue

My dear disciple Huang Di,

It is your teacher, who has been forgotten back into nothingness.

Yes, it is I, the mysterious Lady of the Way, the wisdom that begat the healing of the ages, who whispered the medicine out of the void and into your ear. You knew my life giving spirit in your bones, which your most learned men have killed with the letter.

I sit on the divine white tortoise in my moon palace brewing my elixirs as my ladies prepare the way and breathe me out of hiding.

I feel the quickening; my time is nearing.

Xuan Nu 玄女

Yes, Huang Di, reportedly born through the surge of the spirits, a direct descendent of Shang Di, communed with the goddess. Fierce as dark goddesses often are, she provided an unconventional wisdom that had the power to break through unhealthy systems. This power, like the Valley Spirit, is always with us. It gives birth to children. It has the power to break through barriers and birth new selves. And through you, dear follower of this ancient tradition, it can give birth to a whole new medicine, needed for a whole new earth.

Once female adepts were seen as being ahead of the game in attaining the Way, life-givers had the advantage in birthing the awakened immortal embryo. References to women in Taoism are scant, as their study has been quite neglected. But if we aren't looking to written sources as the only truth, we can follow a thread leading back to the goddess. In some Taoist sects like the southern sacred peak of Nanyue, Lady Wei, once human, attained the Way and became a revered goddess who replaced the deified Xi Wang Mu (Queen Mother of the West). Lady Wei originated many of the Taoist practices for women. Her divine wisdom was received directly, and after her ascendance, she offered the same to her adepts, including Huang Di, who consulted her for guidance and received her transmissions. While we may not be able to "prove" her existence, we haven't proven Huang Di's either.

We are in a time of change where the patriarchal systems of the past do not have what's required to support this new irruptive force. The fathers of medicine have failed us and the hold of the father gods are weakening. There is a changing of the guards and a changing of the gods, and shifting the dominance from information to transformation begins with the life-givers who have learned not to change the outside without first accessing the power of Te within. As channels of this divine mystery, they bow, and remain in astonishment at its wisdom to choose creation as an extension of love, not just survival.

To borrow a metaphor from Abdu'l-Bahá's writings of the Bahá'í faith, the sacred bird of humanity has been flying with a single, masculine, goal-oriented wing for far too long, leaving us circling in mayhem. If we are to survive as a species, the process-oriented wing of the feminine archetype must unfurl, and perhaps we can overcome the limited egoic legacy left by the analytical minds so highly revered by our founding fathers. As we include the tribal knowing deep in our bones, we gain access to another type of wisdom. Like the tailless bird of the Triple Warmer, not meant for flight but for winged transformation, the old must dive into the flames. The divine mother arises from the ashes and rights our course. A new medicine is born. We don't need more healers, but revealers.

Bibliography

Transforming the Void: Embryological Discourse and Reproductive Imagery in East Asian Religions, edited by Anna Andreeva & Dominic Steavu (Brill, 2015)

Chinese Herbal Medicine: Materia Medica, by Dan Bensky, Andrew Gamble, & Ted Kaptchuk (Eastland Press, 1986)

"A model for implantation of the human blastocyst and early placentation," Article by Paul Bischof & Aldo Campana (*Human Reproduction Update 2*(3): 262–270, 1996)

"Treating oligohydramnios with extract of Salvia miltiorrhiza: A randomized control trial," Article by Hong-Nü Chu & Mei-Juan Shen (*Therapeutics and Clinical Risk Management 4*(1): 287–290, 2008)

Immortal Sisters: Secret Teachings of Taoist Women, by Thomas Cleary (North Atlantic Books, 1996)

Five Spirits: Alchemical Acupuncture for Psychological and Spiritual Healing, by Lorie Dechar (Lantern Publishing & Media, 2006)

"A Classical Chinese Medical Perspective on the Nature of Aging and Longevity," Article by Heiner Fruehauf (2010), https://classicalchinesemedicine.org/articles/member-articles

"DNA—the phantom effect, quantum hologram and the etheric body," Article by Linda Gadbois (*MOJ Proteomics & Bioinformatics 7*(1): 9–10. doi:10.15406/mojpb.2018.07.00206, 2018)

The Prophet, by Kahlil Gibran (Alfred A. Knopf, 1923)

Sand and Foam: A Book of Aphorisms, by Kahlil Gibran (Read & Co Books, 2020)

Developmental Biology (8th edn), by Scott F. Gilbert (Sinauer, 2010)

Race and the Cosmos: An Invitation to View the World Differently, by Barbara A. Holmes (Bloomsbury, 2002)

Magical Beginnings, Enchanted Lives, A Guide to Pregnancy and Childbirth, Deepak Chopra, David Simon, Vicki Abrams (Harmony, 2005)

"How the trauma of life is passed down in SPERM, affecting the mental health of future generations," Article by Emma Innes (*Mail Online*, 23 April 2014) (www. dailymail.co.uk/health/article-2611317/How-trauma-life-passed-SPERM-affecting-mental-health-future-generations.html)

MATHNAWI I, 3775-3782 (translated by Kabir Helminski and Camille Helminski)

Guan Zi (Kuan Tzu): The Book of Master Guan Encyclopedia of Chinese Philosophy, Antonio Cua (Routledge, 2003)

Huang Di Nei Jing Ling Shu, by Wu Jing-Nuan (The Taoist Center, 1993)

"Khan Academy, Funeral banner of Lady Dai (Xin Zhui)", (www.khanacademy. org/humanities/ap-art-history/south-east-se-asia/china-art/a/funeral-banner-of-lady-dai-xin-zhui)

The Secret Treatise of the Spiritual Orchid, by Claude Larre (Monkey Press, 2003)

"Animal models of implantation," Article by Kevin Y. Lee & Francisco J. DeMayo (*Reproduction 128*(6): 679–695, 2004)

The Huainanzi: A Guide to the Theory and Practice of Government in Early Han China, by Liu An, King of Huainan (Translations from the Asian Classics), by John S. Major, Sarah A. Queen, Andrew Seth Meyer, & Harold D. Roth (Columbia University Press, 2010)

Soul's Hidden Wholeness, Online Series with Michael Meade (www.mosaicvoices. org/events/souls-hidden-wholeness)

Tao Te Ching, by Stephen Mitchell (HarperCollins, 1999)

The Dance of the Dissident Daughter: A Woman's Journey from Christian Tradition to the Sacred Feminine, by Sue Monk Kidd (HarperCollins Publishers, 2002)

Gnostic Gospels, by Elaine Pagels (Phoenix, 2006)

Power of Place: The Religious Landscape of the Southern Sacred Peak (Nanyue 南嶽) in Medieval China, by James Robson (Harvard University Asia Center, 2009)

Pregnancy and Gestation: In Chinese Classical Texts, by Elizabeth Rochat de la Vallée (Monkey Press, 2007)

"Current studies on human implantation: A brief overview," Article by Peter A.W. Rogers (*Reproduction, Fertility, and Development 7*(6): 1395–1399, 1995)

The Taoist Body, by Kristofer Schipper, Translated by Karen C. Duval (University of California Press, 1993)

Huang Di Nei Jing Su Wen: Nature, Knowledge, Imagery in an Ancient Chinese Medical Text, with an Appendix, the Doctrine of the Five Periods and Six Qi in the Huang Di Nei Jing Su Wen, by Paul U. Unschuld (University of California Press, 2003)

Hua Hu Ching: The Unknown Teachings of Lao Tzu, by Brian Walker (Harper-Collins, 1992)

"Song of Myself, 44," *Leaves of Grass*, Poem by Walt Whitman (1855, https://poets.org/poem/song-myself-44)

The Secret of the Golden Flower: A Chinese Book of Life, by Richard Wilhelm (Harcourt Brace & Co., 1962)

Nurturing the Foetus in Medieval China: Illustrating the 10 Months of Pregnancy in the Ishimpō 醫心方, by Sabine Wilms (Brill, 2018)

Personal lecture notes from Jeffrey Yuen, 2003–2022

Transforming the Void: Embryological Discourse and Reproductive Imagery in East Asian Religions, (Sir Henry Wellcome Asian) Andrea and Steavu, Brill; Lam edition, 2015

Dream Work, Mary Oliver (The Atlantic Monthly Press, 1986)

The oldest medical encyclopedia divided into 50 scrolls, written by court physician Chao Yuanfangwritten during the Sui dynasty (581-618). Learned from lectures given by Jeffrey Yuen, 88th generation Daoist Priest, Jade Purity Tradition, Lao Tau Sect

The Prophet, Kahlil Gibran (Knopf, 1923)

Chuang Tzu Daoist Teachings: Zhuangzi's Wisdom, James Legge, Aziloth, 2017

Zhong He Ji (Qi gong, yang sheng cong shu), Mandarin Chinese Edition, Li Daochun (Shanghai gu ji chu ban she, 1989)

Weidenfeld and Nicolson Response to atheist Alfred Kerr in the winter of 1927, who after deriding ideas of God and religion at a dinner party in the home of the publisher Samuel Fischer, had queried him "I hear that you are supposed to be deeply religious" as quoted in The Diary of a Cosmopolitan (1971) by H. G. Kessler

Biology of Belief, Bruce Lipton (Hay House, 2016)

Secret of the Golden Flower, translated by Richard Wilhelm (Harvest Books, 1962)

St Symeon, The New Theologian (949-1022) from The Center for Action and Contemplation, Prayer of the Heart (December 16, 2021, Richard Rohr)

The Illuminated Rumi, Halal Al-Din Rumi, translated by Coleman Barks, illustrations by Michael Green (Broadway Books, 1997)

Chuang-Tzu: The Inner Chapters (Hackett Classics), Zhuangzi, translated by A.C. Graham (Hacket Publishing Company, UK ed, 2001)

Revelations of Divine Love, Julian of Norwich, translated by Grace Warrack (Independently published, January 2020)

C.G. Jung Psychological Reflections: A New Anthology of His Writings, 1905-1961, C. J. Jung, R.F.C. Hull and Julianne Jacobi, editors, Princeton University Press, Reprint, 1978 (May 1, 1973)